# The Yeast Infection Mastery Bible Your Blueprint For Complete Yeast Infection Management

Dr. Ankita Kashyap and Prof. Krishna N. Sharma

Published by Virtued Press, 2023.

While every precaution has been taken in the preparation of this book, the publisher assumes no responsibility for errors or omissions, or for damages resulting from the use of the information contained herein.

THE YEAST INFECTION MASTERY BIBLE YOUR BLUEPRINT FOR COMPLETE YEAST INFECTION MANAGEMENT

**First edition. November 14, 2023.**

Written by Dr. Ankita Kashyap and Prof. Krishna N. Sharma.

# Table of Contents

# DISCLAIMER

The information provided in this book is intended for general informational purposes only. The content is not meant to substitute professional medical advice, diagnosis, or treatment. Always consult with a qualified healthcare provider before making any changes to your diabetes management plan or healthcare regimen.

While every effort has been made to ensure the accuracy and completeness of the information presented, the author and publisher do not assume any responsibility for errors, omissions, or potential misinterpretations of the content. Individual responses to diabetes management strategies may vary, and what works for one person might not be suitable for another.

The book does not endorse any specific medical treatments, products, or services. Readers are encouraged to seek guidance from their healthcare providers to determine the most appropriate approaches for their unique medical conditions and needs.

Any external links or resources provided in the book are for convenience and informational purposes only. The author and publisher do not have control over the content or availability of these external sources and do not endorse or guarantee the accuracy of such information.

Readers are advised to exercise caution and use their judgment when applying the information provided in this book to their own situations. The author and publisher disclaim any liability for any direct, indirect, consequential, or other damages arising from the use of this book and its content.

By reading and using this book, readers acknowledge and accept the limitations and inherent risks associated with implementing the strategies, recommendations, and information contained herein. It is always recommended to consult a qualified healthcare professional for personalized medical advice and care.

# Introduction

Once upon a time, there was a silent threat hiding in the shadows in a planet teeming with microscopic organisms and microorganisms. This is a voyage into the intricate and enigmatic realm of yeast infections rather than a storey about heroes or villains. Greetings from "The Yeast Infection Mastery Bible: Your Blueprint for Complete Yeast Infection Management" to you, dear reader.

I understand your thoughts at this point. How could yeast infections, such a seemingly uninteresting topic, be fascinating? Hold on to your seats, because I'm going to take you on a fast-paced tour into the human body's microscopic wilderness, where yeast grows and wreaks havoc.

Imagine, if you will, a thriving ecosystem inside of you. Microscopic organisms live in a delicate equilibrium with one another, as friends and foes. Among them, Candida albicans, a cunning little fungus, lurks around, waiting for the right opportunity to strike. Though it might not look like much of a villain, reader, you should not undervalue its power.

But don't worry! Because the key to understanding the mysteries of managing yeast infections is contained inside the pages of this fascinating book. I'm Dr. Ankita Kashyap, a medical professional and health and wellness coach, and I'll be your guide on this trip. And collectively, we will go far into this unusual situation.

I travelled through the maze of reputable medical journals and scientific research as I set out to solve the riddles of yeast infections. Equipped with a pen and an unquenchable curiosity, I explored the very core of this illness, venturing into the furthest reaches of the fields of medicine and complementary and alternative healing.

That's right, reader—where that's the magic is. I have laboriously combined the medical and holistic viewpoints in this well written book to create a symphony of information that will both educate and amuse you. In my search for the truth, I have turned no corner and have accumulated knowledge that is supported by facts to share with you.

I can promise you though, this is not a dry scientific treatise. Instead of falling victim to the dangerous traps of medical language, I have avoided it by using an approachable tone and empathic tone in my writing. You will find yourself casually taking in the material with every page flip, almost like a butterfly delicately fluttering by.

This book is not your average literary work, aye, dear reader. It is an oath to you, my beloved travelling buddy. Every word on every page has been carefully chosen and written to address the particular issues that affect people who have yeast infections.

You will discover a wealth of practical tactics in these sacred pages, all customised to meet your individual requirements. Because this ailment is so varied, I have created individualised strategies and self-help methods that can be tailored to your specific circumstances. Ultimately, no two fights with yeast infections are the same.

For a few minute, picture yourself in a situation where you are in charge of your own health and wellbeing. My dear reader, it is a feasible reality rather than an unrealistic fantasy. By working together, we will be able to control your yeast infection and remove the entanglements that have bound you to it.

So let's get started on this amazing journey right away. Prepare yourself with an open heart, a curious mind, and a dash of whimsy. For there is a wealth of information and empowerment waiting for you inside the pages of "The Yeast Infection Mastery Bible: Your Blueprint for Complete Yeast Infection Management." Start the journey now!

# Chapter 1: Understanding Yeast Infections

# The Science Behind Yeast Infections

# Common Symptoms and Diagnosis

As a medical professional, I have seen a broad spectrum of symptoms in people with yeast infections. While some people could only have one or two symptoms, others might have multiple symptoms combined. It is also important to remember that these symptoms might mimic those of other illnesses, so seeking a medical evaluation from a specialist is crucial.

Itching is the most typical sign of a yeast infection. It might irritate and cause discomfort because it can be strong and persistent. This itching can be more general, affecting the armpits, groyne, or even the mouth in cases of oral thrush, or it can be restricted to the affected location, such as the genital area in cases of vaginal yeast infections.

Inflammation or redness is another typical sign. The afflicted region could seem inflamed, bloated, and red. A thick, white discharge that resembles cottage cheese may be present along with redness and swelling of the vulva and vagina in the event of a vaginal yeast infection.

Regarding discharge, this is another obvious indicator of candida infections. Usually, the discharge is odourless, white, and thick. It could be lumpy or have a cottage cheese-like consistency. While the discharge may occasionally be weak and watery, it usually smells strongly of something other than regular vaginal discharge. When trying to diagnose if the symptoms are coming from a yeast infection or something else entirely, this is a crucial differentiator.

Certain people also feel pain or discomfort when they urinate or have sex. This is due to the possibility that the inflammatory tissues will become sensitive or tender, making pressure or friction painful. It is imperative to get medical assistance for an appropriate diagnosis, as these symptoms may also be suggestive of other illnesses, such as sexually transmitted infections or urinary tract infections.

A rash may also result from a yeast infection in some circumstances. This is more frequently observed in warm, wet regions, such the skin's creases, behind the breasts, or in an infant's diaper area. If treatment is not received, the rash—which is typically red and itchy—may start off as little, raised bumps that spread and worsen. After discussing the typical symptoms, let's examine the diagnostic techniques used by medical specialists to determine the presence of a yeast infection. For proper management and treatment of a yeast infection, a correct diagnosis is essential.

Healthcare providers will often start by taking a complete medical history and performing a physical examination. They will inquire about the nature of your symptoms, when they first appeared, and how they have developed. Inquiries regarding prior yeast infections or other pertinent medical issues may also be made.

The medical professional will visually evaluate the affected area as part of the physical examination. If it's a vaginal yeast infection, they could inspect the cervix using a speculum and collect discharge samples for additional testing. To determine the precise type of yeast causing the infection, these samples can be inspected under a microscope or sent to a lab for culture.

A medical practitioner may also do a "wet mount" test in some circumstances, which entails putting a sample of the vaginal discharge on a slide and looking at it under a microscope. This can assist in determining whether yeast cells are present as well as other possible reasons for the symptoms, like trichomoniasis or bacterial vaginosis.

More tests might be carried out if the symptoms persist or don't go away with conventional therapy. These can include blood testing to look for diseases like diabetes or compromised immune systems that might be causing the yeast infections.

A biopsy is a procedure where a tiny sample of the diseased tissue is surgically removed and studied under a microscope. In certain cases, a healthcare expert may recommend a biopsy. This can confirm the presence of a yeast infection and help rule out other possible explanations of the symptoms.

It is crucial to keep in mind that, despite the widespread use of these diagnostic techniques, a precise diagnosis of yeast infections can occasionally be difficult. This is due to the possibility that distinct people may appear with differing presentations and that the symptoms may be identical to those of other illnesses. For the best course of action when it comes to treating and managing yeast infections, speaking with a medical practitioner who specialises in this area is essential.

In conclusion, being aware of the typical symptoms and indicators of yeast infections can assist people in recognising them and in seeking prompt medical assistance. Typical symptoms include itching, redness, inflammation, abnormal discharge, and discomfort during urination or sexual activity. For a precise diagnosis, it's crucial to speak with a medical expert nevertheless, as there may be overlapping symptoms. Healthcare providers are capable of accurately diagnosing yeast infections and making treatment recommendations based on a patient's medical history, physical examination, and results from additional diagnostic testing.

# Understanding Risk Factors

We will examine the many risk factors that lead to the emergence of yeast infections in this subchapter. Anyone who wants to take control of their health and avoid recurring infections must be aware of these risk factors.

Hormonal Changes:

The development of yeast infections is significantly influenced by hormonal changes. Because their menstrual cycles cause fluctuations in hormone levels, women are particularly vulnerable to these illnesses. Yeast overgrowth may be encouraged in the vaginal region by the increase in oestrogen levels that occurs during ovulation and pregnancy.

Moreover, there may be a higher chance of yeast infections for women using hormonal birth control techniques such hormone-releasing IUDs or oral contraceptives. These methods of birth control have the potential to upset the delicate balance of vaginal flora, which would facilitate the growth of yeast.

Weakened Immune System:

One important additional risk factor for yeast infections is a compromised immune system. Our immune system is essential in the battle against infections, which includes yeast. Nevertheless, a number of things can make it more difficult for the immune system to carry out its defence role.

Diabetes, HIV/AIDS, and autoimmune diseases are examples of chronic illnesses that can impair immune function and increase a person's susceptibility to yeast infections. Additionally, a compromised immune system may result from certain lifestyle choices including poor eating habits, sleep deprivation, and ongoing stress.

Medications:

Moreover, some drugs may make getting a yeast infection more likely. Particularly antibiotics are known to upset the natural flora of the body, giving yeast an opportunity to proliferate. Antibiotics are meant to destroy unwanted bacteria, but they also get rid of good bacteria like lactobacilli, which keep the pH in the vagina ideal.

Additional drugs that have been linked to a higher incidence of yeast infections are immunosuppressants and corticosteroids. These drugs have the potential to weaken the immune system, which makes it more challenging for the body to fight yeast overgrowth.

Diet and Lifestyle Factors:

Yeast infections can also result from particular dietary and lifestyle choices, hormonal changes, immune system deterioration, and drug side effects. Eating a diet high in refined carbs and sugar can provide the yeast the energy it needs to proliferate. Inadequate personal cleanliness and excessive alcohol intake might also foster an atmosphere that is conducive to yeast overgrowth.

Furthermore, wearing clothing that is too tight, especially made of synthetic fabrics, can trap heat and moisture in the vaginal area, which is perfect for yeast growth. Likewise, prolonged exposure to damp swimwear or perspiring exercise attire may heighten the likelihood of developing yeast infections.

Managing yeast infections effectively starts with an understanding of these risk factors. You can reduce your risk of developing yeast infections by being aware of the things that lead to fungal diseases in your own life.

I frequently suggest changing one's lifestyle to control and avoid yeast infections. Modifying one's diet to include less sugar and refined carbohydrates, for example, can help make the atmosphere less conducive to yeast overgrowth. Supplementing the diet with fermented foods or probiotic supplements can also aid in reestablishing the proper balance of good bacteria in the body.

Apart from dietary adjustments, maintaining proper cleanliness is essential to avert yeast infections. This includes refraining from using strong soaps and feminine hygiene products, which may upset the vagina's normal pH balance. Preventing yeast overgrowth can also be achieved by preventing excessive wetness in the vaginal area and wearing breathable cotton underwear.

It could be essential for people with compromised immune systems to take extra care to avoid yeast infections. This could entail treating underlying illnesses proactively, such as diabetes or autoimmune disorders, as well as adopting the right steps to strengthen immunity, such controlling stress levels, eating optimally, and getting enough sleep.

In conclusion, successful therapy and prevention of yeast infections depend on an understanding of the risk factors that lead to their development. People can take charge of their health and lessen the frequency and severity of yeast infections by addressing hormonal shifts, boosting immunity, and adopting appropriate lifestyle modifications. I want to enable people to take charge of their health and find lasting cure from yeast infections through my work as a medical doctor and health and wellness coach.

# Exploring Different Types of Yeast Infections

Understanding the many kinds of yeast infections is crucial as we go deeper into the subject. People must be cognizant of their state because each shape has distinct features and ramifications of its own. Three common forms of yeast infections—oral thrush, systemic yeast infections, and vaginal yeast infections—will be discussed in this chapter.

Vaginal Yeast Infections:

Women of all ages are susceptible to vaginal yeast infections, one of the most common types of yeast infections. Candida albicans is the cause of this ailment; it is a kind of yeast that often lives in the vaginal region. On the other hand, yeast can grow out of control and cause an infection if the delicate balance of microorganisms in the vagina is upset.

A vaginal yeast infection can cause severe itching, redness, swelling, and a thick white discharge, among other symptoms. It is possible for women to feel pain or discomfort when urinating or having sex. If these symptoms increase or persist, you should contact a doctor because a correct diagnosis is necessary for a successful course of therapy.

Oral Thrush:

Oral candidiasis, another name for oral thrush, is a yeast infection that affects the throat and mouth. People with compromised immune systems—such as those receiving chemotherapy, taking immunosuppressive drugs, or living with HIV/AIDS—are more likely to experience this illness. Oral thrush is also more common in young children, the elderly, and those with diabetes.

Creamy white lesions on the tongue, inner cheeks, gums, tonsils, or back of the throat are the most noticeable sign of oral thrush. When scraped, these sores may bleed and cause pain. In extreme situations, people could also have trouble swallowing or feel like they have cotton in their mouths. In order to reduce symptoms and stop the infection from spreading, therapy must be started as away.

Systemic Yeast Infections:

Oral thrush and vaginal yeast infections are localised conditions, but systemic yeast infections are significantly more dangerous and can impact multiple organs and systems across the body. This kind of infection, also called candidemia, happens when yeast enters the bloodstream and travels to other parts of the body, like the brain, heart, or lungs.

Systemic yeast infections are more common in those with compromised immune systems, such as those with HIV/AIDS, undergoing organ transplantation, or in critical care. Even those with good immune systems, however, may become ill with this condition, particularly if they have recently had certain medical operations done or have been on long-term antibiotic therapy.

Depending on which organs are impacted, systemic yeast infections can cause a variety of symptoms, such as fever, chills, fast heartbeat, disorientation, and organ failure. Seeking medical help right away is imperative if you think you may have a systemic yeast infection. Timely diagnosis and targeted treatment are critical for optimal results.

Understanding the Implications:

Yeast infections can be considered a minor inconvenience, but there are serious consequences that can affect a person's general health and well-being. Beyond the discomfort and physical symptoms, recurrent yeast infections can negatively influence a person's quality of life by impairing relationships, self-esteem, and everyday functioning.

In addition, problems may arise from untreated or persistent yeast infections. Recurrence of vaginal yeast infections, for instance, can harm the delicate vaginal tissues, resulting in inflammation, persistent pain, and heightened vulnerability to other infections. Furthermore, untreated systemic yeast infections have the ability to spread and seriously harm organs, possibly even posing a life-threatening hazard.

Thus, it is critical to address and prevent the consequences linked to yeast infections through early diagnosis, adequate medication, and comprehensive management. Through providing individuals with information regarding the many forms of yeast infections and their consequences, we facilitate proactive health management and overall well-being.

We will examine the causes, risk factors, diagnosis techniques, and efficacious treatment options of each type of yeast infection in more detail in the upcoming chapters. We will also examine the relationship between yeast infections and other underlying medical issues, providing insight into the interactions that occur between our immune systems, bodies, and candida overgrowth.

People may take back control of their health, fostering harmony within their bodies and feeling rejuvenated, by learning everything there is to know about yeast infections and how to treat them. I'd want to ask you to embrace the transformational power of information as we go on this journey together and start down the path to mastery over yeast infections.

# Chapter 2: Medical Management of Yeast Infections

# Antifungal Medications and Treatments

Selecting the appropriate course of action for yeast infections is critical to their successful management. Thankfully, there are a number of antifungal drugs and therapies that can assist in reducing the symptoms and clearing the body of the underlying fungal infection. We will examine the available options, their efficacy, possible drawbacks, and usage instructions in this subsection so that you can choose your course of treatment with knowledge.

1. Topical Antifungal Medications:

When treating yeast infections, topical antifungal drugs are frequently the first line of treatment. These drugs are administered topically to the afflicted area as creams, ointments, lotions, or suppositories. They function by eradicating the yeast or preventing its growth, which also relieves symptoms like swelling, redness, and itching.

Clotrimazole is one of the topical antifungal drugs that is most frequently administered. The majority of yeast infections can be successfully treated with this over-the-counter drug. Usually, it is used once or twice a day for a few days, or until the symptoms go away.

Miconazole is another well-liked option that may be purchased over-the-counter. It is administered directly to the afflicted area, just like clotrimazole, and is usually used for seven to ten days. The adverse effects of both miconazole and clotrimazole are thought to be insignificant and include some burning or irritation at the application site.

For severe or recurring yeast infections, prescription-strength topical antifungal drugs such ketoconazole or econazole may be advised. These drugs may need a longer course of treatment because they are often stronger. To guarantee that your medication is working as intended, it's critical that you adhere to your doctor's recommendations and finish the entire prescribed course.

2. Oral Antifungal Medications:

Oral antifungal drugs may be used if topical therapies are ineffective or if the yeast infection is more extensive. By eliminating the fungus from within the body, these drugs are able to reach places that topical treatments are unable to.

One of the oral antifungal drugs that is most frequently recommended is fluconazole. It is often administered as a single dose and is quite efficient against yeast infections. After taking the prescription as directed, the symptoms typically start to get better a few days later. However, it's crucial to keep taking the medication as directed until the entire course is finished.

Although oral antifungal drugs are generally well tolerated and safe, there are a few possible side effects to be mindful of. These could include headaches, diarrhoea, nausea, and abdominal pain. Rarely, more severe side effects like liver damage may manifest, therefore it's critical to notify your healthcare professional right away if you experience any strange symptoms.

3. Alternative and Complementary Treatments:

To support the management of yeast infections, complementary and alternative therapies can be employed in addition to traditional antifungal drugs. For milder cases, these treatments are frequently used alone or in conjunction with conventional drugs.

Probiotics, which are good bacteria that aid in reestablishing the body's natural microbiological equilibrium, are one such treatment. Probiotics can be applied topically as creams or suppositories, or they can be consumed as supplements. They can support the maintenance of a healthy vaginal environment and help stop the overgrowth of yeast.

Boric acid is another possible therapy approach. Studies have demonstrated the efficaciousness of boric acid suppositories in treating recurring yeast infections, particularly those resulting from non-albicans yeast species. But since boric acid can be hazardous if taken improperly, it should only be used under a doctor's supervision.

Herbal medications with natural antifungal qualities, such tea tree oil or oregano oil, are other complementary therapies that might be helpful in managing yeast infections. It's crucial to remember that these medications can irritate some people or trigger allergic responses, so they should only be used sparingly and under a doctor's supervision.

4. Lifestyle Modifications and Self-Care Techniques:

Changing one's lifestyle and adopting self-care habits can be very helpful in controlling yeast infections, in addition to pharmaceutical and complementary therapies.

Keeping oneself clean is crucial. Avoid wearing tight clothes or synthetic underwear, which can trap moisture and encourage the growth of yeast, and keep the afflicted region dry and clean. Instead, go with breathable cotton panties.

The use of strong soaps, douches, or perfumed products in the vaginal area should also be avoided because they might irritate the sensitive tissues and upset the natural balance. Alternatively, use gentle, fragrance-free cleaners or only warm water to clean.

A balanced diet low in processed foods and sugar can help avoid yeast overgrowth and strengthen the immune system. Foods high in probiotics, such kefir and yoghurt, can also help to keep the vaginal flora healthy.

Stress can lead to yeast infections, therefore practising stress-reduction strategies like yoga, deep breathing, or meditation can help lower stress levels. The immune system as a whole can also be supported by frequent exercise, eating a healthy weight, and obtaining adequate sleep.

In summary, a variety of antifungal drugs and therapies are available to treat yeast infections, each having unique advantages and drawbacks. Whether you choose oral or topical drugs, complementary therapies, or lifestyle changes, it's crucial to speak with a healthcare professional to figure out which course of action is best for your particular circumstances. You can successfully manage and avoid recurrent infections, guaranteeing long-term relief and general well-being, by treating the yeast infection comprehensively and addressing its underlying cause.

# Preventive Measures and Hygiene Practices

Let's first create a clear grasp of yeast infections before getting into the intricacies. The overgrowth of the Candida fungus, primarily Candida albicans, is the cause of yeast infections, sometimes referred to as candidiasis. Our bodies naturally contain this fungus, usually in the mouth, vagina, and gastrointestinal system. However, the yeast can grow and result in an infection in some situations, such as when the body's natural microflora is out of balance or when the immune system is weakened.

Although they mostly affect the vaginal or penile area in men and women, respectively, yeast infections are frequent in both sexes. The symptoms, which can include burning, itching, redness, and an unusual discharge, can be upsetting and painful. One's quality of life may be greatly impacted by recurring yeast infections, which can cause annoyance, self-consciousness, and even low self-esteem.

What can we do, then, to stop these infections before they start? The solution is to maintain the delicate balance of bacteria in our bodies by maintaining excellent hygiene and taking preventative measures.

In order to lower the risk of yeast infections, proper genital cleanliness is crucial. This includes cleaning the vaginal region with water and mild, fragrance-free soap for women. Douching or using harsh chemical products must be avoided as they can upset the vagina's natural pH balance and perhaps cause an overgrowth of yeast. Furthermore, always remember to wipe from front to back after using the restroom to stop bacteria and yeast from moving from the anus to the vaginal area.

Men should wash their penis and surrounding area every day with warm water and a mild soap as part of good genital hygiene. Similar to what happens with women, keeping a healthy balance of microorganisms in the genital area depends on avoiding harsh chemical products and making sure the area is completely dried after bathing.

Selecting breathable clothing is another preventive step people can take to lower their chance of developing yeast infections. It is essential to wear clothing made of natural materials that promote air circulation, such cotton, since yeast grows best in warm, damp situations. Keeping the vaginal area dry and uninviting for yeast overgrowth can also be achieved by avoiding tight-fitting jeans or underwear that could trap moisture and heat.

Because certain irritants might raise the likelihood of yeast infections, it is equally vital to be cautious of the things we use on our bodies. This covers scented laundry detergents, bubble baths, feminine hygiene products, and even soaps. These items frequently include chemicals and scents that might cause an overgrowth of yeast in our systems and upset the natural equilibrium of our bodies. Choosing hypoallergenic, fragrance-free products can help lower this risk.

Establishing general hygiene routines is also essential to maintaining a healthy lifestyle. To stop the transmission of germs and yeast from outside sources, such polluted surfaces or items, this involves routinely washing your hands. Do not share personal goods with other people, including washcloths or towels, in order to reduce the possibility of spreading bacteria or yeast.

Including a healthy, balanced diet that promotes gut health is another prophylactic that can drastically lower the incidence of yeast infections. Yogurt, kefir, sauerkraut, and other fermented foods are high in probiotics, which can support a balanced population of bacteria in the body. Probiotics are good microorganisms that can prevent Candida overgrowth and assist in preserving the ideal pH balance.

Practicing self-care practises and managing stress are essential in lowering the incidence of yeast infections, in addition to dietary modifications. The immune system can be weakened by stress, increasing the body's vulnerability to infections. Deep breathing exercises, yoga, meditation, and other relaxation techniques can all help reduce stress and enhance general wellbeing. Maintaining a healthy weight, getting adequate sleep, and exercising frequently are all essential for fostering the best possible immune system performance.

Finally, it's critical to understand the variables that could raise the chance of developing a yeast infection. Antibiotics, for instance, have the ability to upset the body's normal microbial balance, which may result in an overabundance of yeast. If you receive an antibiotic prescription, talk to your doctor about the potential to reduce this risk by taking probiotics both during and after treatment.

Furthermore, those with compromised immune systems or underlying medical disorders like diabetes are more prone to recurring yeast infections. If this describes you, you should collaborate closely with your physician to create a thorough strategy that takes care of the underlying issue as well as preventative steps against yeast infections.

In summary, avoiding yeast infections involves a multifaceted strategy that emphasises self-care, lifestyle changes, and proper cleanliness. You may considerably lower your risk of developing yeast infections and experience an improvement in your general health by adopting these preventive steps into your everyday routine. Always keep in mind that prevention is the key to controlling yeast infections. With the appropriate information and a proactive mindset, you may attain optimal health and be free from the discomfort of recurring infections.

# Partner Management and Prevention

It is important to realise that sexual contact can be a means of transmission for yeast infections. If a person receives a diagnosis of yeast infection, it's critical to discuss the condition with their spouse. While some people may find this uncomfortable, it is necessary for both parties' well-being and to stop reinfection. In every partnership, communication that is honest and open is essential, especially when it comes to health-related issues.

Transmission Risk:

Transmission of yeast infections can happen during close sexual contact, such as anal, oral, or vaginal sex. Although there is a greater chance of transmission when one partner has an active yeast infection, the infection can still spread even in the absence of symptoms. This is due to the fact that yeast may survive on mucous membranes and skin, upsetting the delicate balance of bacteria.

Safe Sexual Practices:

It is essential to practise safe sexual activities in order to reduce the chance of transmission. One strategy is to utilise barrier techniques like condoms or dental dams consistently and correctly. These physical barriers can lessen the spread of yeast between couples and help avoid direct skin-to-skin contact.

Keeping yourself clean is a crucial part of healthy sexual behaviour. Before engaging in sexual activity, it is advised to cleanse the vaginal area with water and mild, unscented soap. Urinating before and after sexual activity is something that both couples should think about doing to assist clear the urethra of any bacteria that may have gotten within.

Treatment Considerations for Partners:

It's critical to treat a yeast infection in one partner with consideration for the other partner. It is important to examine both people for yeast infections and treat them appropriately if needed. If the afflicted partner is the only one receiving treatment, this could lead to a reinfection cycle in which the infection alternates between partners.

If a yeast infection is discovered in both partners, it is advised to wait to engage in sexual activity until after each partner has finished treatment and their symptoms have subsided. This will enable both people to recuperate completely and help prevent reinfection.

It's crucial to talk about treatment choices when one partner is diagnosed with a yeast infection even when they don't exhibit any symptoms. In order to protect against reinfection and to guarantee the health of both parties, certain medical specialists could advise treating the asymptomatic spouse. A healthcare professional should be consulted before making this choice.

Partner Support and Communication:

In order to control yeast infections in a partnership, communication must be transparent and sincere. It is crucial that both parties offer understanding and emotional support throughout this period. A supportive and listening partner can play a crucial role in aiding the healing process of yeast infections, which can lead to discomfort, agony, and mental distress.

The relationship between people can also be strengthened by encouraging partners to participate in the treatment plan. This can entail going to doctor's visits with the afflicted partner, doing joint research and education on yeast infections, and collaborating to adopt healthy lifestyle modifications.

Prevention Strategies:

It is usually better to avoid yeast infections in the first place rather than manage the symptoms and therapy. The following techniques will lessen the likelihood of getting a yeast infection:

1. Practice good hygiene: Avoid using scented products or douches, which can upset the natural balance of bacteria, and keep the genital area dry and clean.

2. Wear breathable clothing: Choose loose-fitting clothes that can retain moisture and foster an atmosphere that is conducive to yeast proliferation, and stick to cotton underwear instead.

3. Avoid excessive moisture: After working out or swimming, change out of your damp clothes right away, and make sure your genital area is completely dry.

4. Choose the right lubricants: Water-based lubricants are better than silicone- or oil-based lubricants because the latter can harbour yeast.

5. Maintain a healthy lifestyle: Stronger immunity and general wellness can be attributed to a balanced diet, consistent exercise, enough sleep, and stress reduction.

6. Limit antibiotic use: Avoid using antibiotics when not essential as they can upset the body's natural balance of microbes.

By putting these preventative techniques into practise and engaging in safe sexual conduct, people can lower their risk of getting a yeast infection and safeguard their partners' and their own health.

To sum up, effective partner management and prevention techniques are essential for controlling and averting yeast infections. A holistic approach to managing yeast infections must include open and honest conversation, safe sexual conduct, and therapeutic consideration for both couples. Healthy intimate relationships can be maintained and the chance of reinfection can be reduced by putting prevention techniques into practise and helping one another through the healing process. Never forget that the goal of managing a yeast infection should always be the health and happiness of both partners.

# Recurrent Yeast Infections and Treatment Options

Understanding Recurrent Yeast Infections:

Four or more vaginal yeast infection episodes in a year are considered recurrent yeast infections, also called recurrent vulvovaginal candidiasis. Recurrent yeast infections present a greater difficulty than infrequent ones, which are common and easily treatable. The symptoms, which can be extremely uncomfortable and recurrent and include burning, itching, redness, and a thick, white discharge, can be experienced by people who are impacted.

Understanding the fundamental causes of this illness is crucial to gaining deeper insights. Candida albicans is the most prevalent cause of recurring yeast infections. This type of fungus naturally exists in the vagina in modest amounts. However, Candida albicans can overgrow and cause an infection if the delicate balance of the vaginal ecology is upset. This imbalance can be caused by a number of things, including:

1. Hormonal Fluctuations: The pH of the vagina can alter due to hormonal changes that occur throughout the menstrual cycle, pregnancy, or menopause, which can lead to an environment that is favourable for yeast overgrowth.

2. Antibiotic Use: While antibiotics are useful in the treatment of bacterial infections, they can also upset the normal balance of bacteria in the vagina, increasing the risk of yeast overgrowth.

3. Weakened Immune System: While antibiotics are useful in the treatment of bacterial infections, they can also upset the normal balance of bacteria in the vagina, increasing the risk of yeast overgrowth.

4. Uncontrolled Diabetes: An environment that encourages the growth of yeast can be created by high blood sugar, which increases the risk of recurring yeast infections in people with uncontrolled diabetes.

5. Personal Hygiene Products: Detergents, strong soaps, and feminine hygiene items can upset the balance in the vaginal environment and increase the risk of recurring yeast infections.

Exploring Alternative Treatment Options:

Conventional antifungal drugs are successful in treating yeast infections, but they might not be a long-term solution for people who get infections frequently. This is the point at which looking into alternate therapy choices becomes essential. People can drastically lower the frequency and severity of recurring yeast infections by using a comprehensive strategy that treats the underlying causes of the infection in addition to its symptoms. Here are a few other therapy alternatives you might want to think about:

1. Probiotics: When ingested, probiotics—live microorganisms—offer health benefits. Research has demonstrated that some probiotic strains, like Lactobacillus acidophilus and Lactobacillus rhamnosus, can assist in reestablishing the normal bacterial balance in the vagina, which lowers the risk of recurring yeast infections. Including foods and pills high in probiotics in your diet could be a helpful complement to your treatment plan.

2. Herbal Remedies: Numerous herbs possess antifungal qualities that can aid in the fight against yeast infections. For instance, studies have demonstrated the antifungal efficacy of tea tree oil against Candida albicans. It is crucial to remember that some herbal medicines have the potential to irritate the skin or trigger allergic reactions, so it is best to speak with a healthcare provider before taking them.

3. Lifestyle Modifications: The chance of recurring yeast infections can be considerably reduced by implementing specific lifestyle modifications. Simple yet effective ways to maintain a healthy vaginal environment include wearing loose-fitting clothing, avoiding perfumed feminine hygiene products, and maintaining proper personal cleanliness.

4. Stress Management: Prolonged anxiety impairs immunity, increasing the body's susceptibility to infections, particularly yeast infections. Including stress-reduction strategies like yoga, meditation, or taking up a hobby can boost general wellbeing and lower stress levels.

5. Dietary Modifications: Dietary changes may help prevent recurring yeast infections, according to some study. A healthy vaginal environment may be supported by limiting sugar and refined carbohydrate intake, which can feed yeast, and concentrating instead on a diet high in whole grains, fruits, vegetables, and lean proteins.

It is important to remember that even while these alternative treatment approaches seem promising in treating recurrent yeast infections, speaking with a healthcare provider is necessary to ascertain which course of action is best for each individual. A customised treatment plan based on a thorough evaluation of your medical history, lifestyle, and general health will be developed.

In Conclusion,

Recurrent yeast infections necessitate a multifaceted strategy that extends beyond prescription drugs. People can take charge of their health and find long-lasting relief from the bothersome symptoms and recurrent yeast infection burdens by learning about the underlying causes and investigating alternate treatment choices. My goal is for this chapter to act as a guide for readers as they work through the difficulties of dealing with recurring yeast infections, leading them to total control over their condition and an enhanced quality of life.

# Chapter 3: Holistic Approaches to Yeast Infection Management

# Dietary Modifications and Yeast Infections

We are used to eating a diet high in processed foods, refined sugars, and harmful fats in today's society. Unfortunately, yeast loves this kind of diet because it creates the ideal conditions for its growth. One kind of fungus that is found naturally in human bodies is yeast, namely Candida albicans. But when our gut's bacterial balance is off, yeast can grow and produce a host of symptoms, such as pain, inflammation, and itching.

Foods that encourage yeast overgrowth should be avoided, as this is one of the most important dietary adjustments for people with yeast infections. Typically, these foods are heavy in sugars, yeast, and processed carbs. It's crucial to remember that, even while a brief withdrawal from these meals could be essential, complete avoidance isn't always necessary. Maintaining a healthy gut flora and bringing the body back into equilibrium are the objectives.

Some of the foods that should be avoided include:

1. Sugary foods and beverages: Since yeast feeds on sugar, you must restrict your consumption of sweets, sugar-filled beverages, and processed snacks. Candies, drinks, pastries, and desserts fall within this category.

2. Refined carbohydrates: Yeast overgrowth can also be facilitated by foods manufactured with white flour, such as crackers, white bread, and pasta. Rather, choose whole grain substitutes.

3. Fermented foods: Although foods that have undergone fermentation have been shown to provide health benefits, they should be avoided in the early stages of managing a yeast infection due to their high yeast content. Foods like kimchi, sauerkraut, and some varieties of cheese fall under this category.

4. Alcohol: In addition to being heavy in sugar, alcohol can upset the delicate balance of gut flora. While treating a yeast infection, limit or stay away from alcohol consumption.

5. Dairy products: Dairy products, especially those high in lactose, may make some people's symptoms of yeast infection worse. Try cutting back on or eliminating dairy from your diet to see if that helps with your symptoms.

After discussing things to stay away from, let's move on to healthy eating adjustments. The objectives of these modifications are to lessen inflammation, boost the immune system, and bring the gut microbiota back into balance. The following dietary suggestions will significantly help you control your yeast infection:

1. Anti-inflammatory foods: Eating a diet high in anti-inflammatory foods can help lower inflammation and alleviate the symptoms of a yeast infection. Berries, leafy greens, ginger, turmeric, and fatty seafood like salmon and mackerel are a few examples.

2. Probiotic-rich foods: Foods high in probiotics, such as kefir, sauerkraut, and yoghurt, can help heal the gut by bringing good bacteria back into balance. In certain circumstances, probiotic pills might also be helpful.

3. Fiber-rich foods: Eating a diet high in fibre can assist in preventing constipation, which can exacerbate yeast overgrowth, and maintaining regular bowel movements. Nuts, fruits, vegetables, whole grains, and legumes are a few foods high in fibre.

4. Antioxidant-rich foods: Antioxidants strengthen the immune system as a whole and help fight oxidative stress. Eat a diet rich in foods like dark chocolate, almonds, green tea, and colourful fruits and vegetables.

5. Hydration: Maintaining a healthy gut and general health depend on drinking enough water. Make it a point to stay hydrated throughout the day to aid in your body's natural cleansing procedures.

6. Balanced macronutrients: Make an effort to include protein, fats, and carbohydrates in your meals in a balanced manner. This encourages satiety, keeps blood sugar levels steady, and gives your body the energy it needs.

Apart from dietary adjustments, it's crucial to take gut health into account when addressing yeast overgrowth. Trillions of bacteria and other microorganisms make up the gut microbiome, which is essential for preserving general health. Dysbiosis, or an imbalance of the gut microbiome, can result from a disturbance in the balance of bacteria in the gut.

Many things, including an unhealthy diet, stress, drugs, and pollutants in the environment, can lead to dysbiosis. Yeast can grow when dysbiosis is present and cause a number of health problems, including yeast infections. Thus, maintaining and improving gut health is crucial for managing yeast infections.

There are several strategies that can be implemented to improve gut health:

1. Probiotics: Live microorganisms known as probiotics have the ability to regulate the gut flora. Think about including items high in probiotics in your diet or using a high-quality probiotic supplement.

2. Prebiotics: Prebiotics are fibres that provide nourishment to the good bacteria in the stomach. Including foods high in prebiotics, such onions, garlic, bananas, and asparagus, can promote the growth of good bacteria in the body.

3. Stress management: Gut health can be adversely affected by ongoing stress. Include stress-reduction strategies in your everyday routine, such as frequent exercise, deep breathing exercises, and meditation.

4. Avoid unnecessary medications: The equilibrium of microorganisms in the stomach can be upset by antibiotics in particular. Use antibiotics sparingly, and when appropriate, collaborate with your healthcare physician to look into other treatments.

5. Detoxification: Toxins that may aggravate dysbiosis can be removed with the help of the body's natural detoxification processes. This can be accomplished by maintaining a healthy diet, getting regular exercise, and drinking enough water.

In summary, dietary changes are essential for managing yeast infections. By removing foods that encourage yeast overgrowth and implementing healthy dietary adjustments, people can assist their body's inherent healing mechanisms and reduce symptoms. Furthermore, improving gut health via methods like probiotic supplements, stress reduction, and detoxification can increase the efficacy of treating yeast infections. Never forget that seeking medical advice is always necessary before implementing any major dietary adjustments or beginning a new supplement regimen.

# Herbal Remedies and Supplements

As a holistic medical professional, I genuinely think that natural treatments and vitamins can help manage yeast infections. This chapter will cover the potential health advantages of a variety of supplements and herbal medicines, such as garlic, tea tree oil, probiotics, and more. When treating yeast infections, these natural remedies can be a mild but effective solution that doesn't have the negative side effects of many prescription drugs.

1. Probiotics: Nature's Healthy Bacteria

Probiotics are good bacteria that are essential for preserving the proper balance of microorganisms within the body. They work particularly well for treating yeast infections brought on by an unbalanced vaginal flora. Probiotics can help stop the overgrowth of Candida, the fungus that causes the majority of yeast infections, by reestablishing the normal balance of microorganisms in the body.

Studies have demonstrated the antifungal characteristics of several probiotic strains, including Lactobacillus acidophilus and Lactobacillus rhamnosus. These probiotics generate compounds that prevent Candida from growing and adhering, hence lowering the likelihood of recurring yeast infections. Probiotics can also boost immunity, which improves the body's capacity to fend against illnesses.

You can add probiotics to your treatment of yeast infections by supplementing with a high-quality product that contains these good bacteria. Seek for a product with a high colony-forming unit (CFU) count and a variety of strains. Selecting a probiotic that is especially designed for vaginal health is also crucial. Lactobacillus crispatus and Lactobacillus plantarum strains, which are very helpful for preserving the balance of vaginal flora, are frequently included in these supplements.

2. Garlic: Nature's Antibacterial and Antifungal Superhero

For generations, people have turned to garlic as a natural cure for a range of illnesses, including yeast infections. Allicin, a substance found in it, has strong antifungal and antibacterial effects. Garlic is a great complement to your plan for managing yeast infections because of these qualities.

Garlic has been shown in numerous studies to have antifungal properties against various species of Candida. By rupturing the fungus's cell membrane and reducing the function of its enzymes, it can stop its growth. Additionally, garlic strengthens the immune system, making the body more capable of fending off illnesses.

You can apply garlic directly to the affected area or take it orally to reap its benefits. While some people would rather take supplements containing garlic, others would rather consume raw garlic. Crush a clove of raw garlic and let it aside for a few minutes to release the allicin. After that, you can use it as a vaginal wash by diluting it in warm water or adding it to your meals. It's crucial to remember that using garlic topically for an extended period of time or in excess can irritate the skin, so it's best to speak with a doctor before attempting this treatment.

3. Tea Tree Oil: Nature's Soothing Antifungal Agent

The antifungal qualities of tea tree oil, which is extracted from the leaves of the Melaleuca alternifolia tree, are widely recognised. Terpinen-4-ol, a substance found in it, has potent antifungal activity against Candida species. Because of this, tea tree oil works well as a natural treatment for yeast infections.

Studies have demonstrated that by rupturing the cell membrane of Candida albicans and disrupting its enzyme function, tea tree oil can stop the fungus from growing. Additionally, it can provide calming relief by lowering the burning, itching, and inflammation brought on by yeast infections.

Use a few drops of pure, therapeutic-grade tea tree oil diluted in a carrier oil, like coconut or olive oil, to treat yeast infections. A few times a day, apply the mixture to the affected area, being careful not to get any on delicate skin or mucous membranes. Before applying tea tree oil topically, you must undergo a patch test to be sure you won't have any negative side effects. Should you encounter any irritation, stop using it right once and seek medical advice.

4. Oregano Oil: Nature's Natural Antimicrobial

The leaves of the Origanum vulgare plant are used to make oregano oil, which has strong antibacterial properties due to the presence of chemicals like thymol and carvacrol. Oregano oil is a useful complement to your yeast infection treatment regimen because of these ingredients, which can aid in the fight against fungal overgrowth.

Studies have shown that by rupturing the cell membranes of Candida species and reducing their enzyme activity, oregano oil can successfully stop their growth. Additionally, it has immune-boosting qualities that help the body fight off infections.

Apply a few drops of oregano oil topically to the afflicted region after diluting it with a carrier oil to treat yeast infections. Because oregano oil can irritate skin when applied topically, it is essential to dilute it. As an alternative, you can consume liquid drops or capsules containing oregano oil orally. But it's imperative that you adhere to the manufacturer's suggested dosage guidelines or seek advice from a medical expert.

5. Calendula: Nature's Soothing and Healing Flower

Due to its calming and restorative qualities, calendula, commonly known as marigold, has been used in traditional medicine for generations. Because it includes substances that have anti-inflammatory, antibacterial, and antifungal properties, it's a great natural treatment for yeast infections.

Calendula has been found to disrupt the cellular structures of Candida and other fungi, hence inhibiting their growth. Additionally, it has the ability to heal wounds by lowering inflammation and encouraging the regeneration of injured tissues.

You can topically apply calendula cream or ointment to the affected region to maximise its advantages. This may lessen the burning, itching, and swelling brought on by yeast infections. Calendula-infused oils or teas can also be used as an all-natural cleanse for the afflicted area. But it's crucial to remember that calendula may cause allergies in certain people, so it's best to do a patch test before using it frequently.

Conclusion:

A natural and gentle way to treat this frequent problem is to include supplements and herbal medicines in your management strategy for yeast infections. Calendula, tea tree oil, garlic, probiotics, and oregano oil are just a handful of the numerous natural substitutes that are out there. But keep in mind that every person may react differently, and these solutions shouldn't take the place of medical advice or care from a specialist. Prior to include any new vitamins or treatments in your regimen, always get advice from a licenced healthcare professional.

The importance that nutrition and diet play in managing yeast infections will be covered in the upcoming chapter, along with a discussion of the best foods to eat in order to support your body's natural defences against yeast overgrowth. Watch this space for insightful commentary and useful advice on assisting your holistic path to total control of yeast infections.

# Stress Management and Emotional Well-being

I am a physician and a health and wellness coach, and I genuinely think that general health is greatly influenced by the mind-body link. Stress can exacerbate symptoms of yeast infections and slow down the healing process. In addition to reducing symptoms, addressing stress head-on strengthens the immune system and expedites the healing process.

Stress management is greatly aided by the use of relaxation techniques. They can aid in lowering stress and fostering serenity and wellbeing. Deep breathing is one such method. Through deliberate attention to our breathing and the practise of deep, calm breathing, we trigger the relaxation response in our bodies. This method aids in lowering blood pressure, heart rate, and cortisol levels—the stress hormone that causes inflammation and exacerbates yeast infections.

Progressive muscle relaxation has also received a lot of attention lately as a relaxing method (PMR). To attain a state of relaxation, PMR entails methodically tensing and then relaxing each muscle group in the body. Stress can be effectively reduced and a sense of physical and mental well-being can be fostered by bringing awareness to our bodies and consciously releasing tension.

Additionally essential to stress management and improving emotional well-being are mindfulness exercises. Being totally present and judgment-free in the moment is a key component of mindfulness. By engaging in mindfulness practises, we can develop a stronger sense of self-awareness and be fully present in our activities, as opposed to being overcome by stress and anxiety.

Meditation is a highly effective mindfulness technique. Through meditation, we can develop inner peace, quiet the mind, and relax the nervous system. It has been demonstrated to lessen sadness, anxiety, and stress—all of which can make yeast infections worse. Frequent meditation practise can improve mental clarity, emotional health, and general quality of life.

Managing stress and fostering emotional well-being need us to integrate coping mechanisms into our everyday lives. Coping mechanisms can assist us in resiliency and adaptation when navigating difficult circumstances. A method that works well is journaling. Writing down our ideas and emotions helps us to become more self-aware, free ourselves from emotional weights, and obtain clarity. Writing in a journal can be a therapeutic exercise that gives us a secure, accepting environment in which to share our feelings.

Another coping mechanism that is highly beneficial for stress management and mental wellbeing is exercise. The "feel-good" hormones, or endorphins, are released by our bodies when we exercise. These endorphins enhance mood, lessen stress, and promote general wellbeing. Exercise on a regular basis can help strengthen our immune system, which is important while fighting yeast infections.

Using a holistic approach is crucial for managing stress and maintaining mental health. This entails taking into account a range of factors including our lifestyle, nutrition, relationships, and self-care routines that affect our general well-being. In order to properly manage stress and promote emotional well-being, self-care must be prioritised.

Activities that nourish and refresh our mind, body, and spirit are included in self-care practises. This can involve taking care of ourselves, pampering ourselves, pursuing hobbies, going outside, practising self-compassion, and taking part in joyful and fulfilling activities. Making self-care a priority lays a solid basis for stress management, emotional health enhancement, and general quality of life improvement.

In summary, emotional stability and stress reduction are essential elements in managing yeast infections. Through the application of mindfulness practises, relaxation techniques, and coping skills, we can successfully mitigate stress and expedite the healing process.

Furthermore, embracing a holistic strategy that includes self-care techniques promotes mental, physical, and spiritual well-being. Long-term improvement of general health and well-being as well as the management of yeast infections depend on stress reduction and emotional stability.

# Exploring Alternative Therapies

For millennia, acupuncture has been utilised as a traditional Chinese medicine to support bodily balance and well-being. In order to promote energy flow and bring balance back to the body, tiny needles are inserted into designated spots. Although the thought of having needles inserted into your skin may be unsettling, acupuncture is a gentle and efficient treatment that offers several advantages to people with yeast infections.

Studies have demonstrated that acupuncture can help control inflammation and the immune system, both of which are critical in lowering the frequency and severity of yeast infections. Acupuncture can also assist in balancing hormones, which in certain cases may be a cause in recurrent yeast infections. Acupuncture helps enhance general well-being by supporting the body's inherent defences against yeast infections by correcting underlying imbalances in the body.

Another complementary therapy that may be helpful in managing yeast infections is homoeopathy. The foundation of homoeopathy is the idea of "like heals like," which states that a drug that causes symptoms in a healthy individual can be administered in tiny quantities to treat the same symptoms in an ill individual. Homeopathic treatments for yeast infections are safe and side effect-free because they are derived from naturally occurring materials and are extremely diluted.

Homeopathy provides a range of medicines for managing yeast infections that can be customised to meet the unique symptoms and requirements of each patient. These treatments function by igniting the body's defences and encouraging self-healing. For instance, to boost the body's defences against the infection, a homoeopathic treatment prepared from the Candida fungus itself may be applied. Some treatments could focus on particular symptoms like burning, itching, or discharge.

A holistic approach to medicine, naturopathy aims to find and treat the underlying causes of illness. A patient's physical, mental, and emotional health are considered by naturopathic doctors when creating a treatment plan. A naturopathic approach to yeast infections may include dietary adjustments, herbal therapies, and lifestyle changes.

Nutrition is a key factor in managing yeast infections, and naturopathic physicians frequently suggest a low-sugar, anti-inflammatory diet to bolster the body's defences against excessive yeast growth. To support a healthy gut flora, this may entail limiting sugar, refined carbs, and processed foods and consuming foods and supplements high in probiotics. Garlic and oregano oil are examples of herbal therapies that can be used to help eliminate excess yeast from the body.

A key component of naturopathic yeast infection treatment is changing one's lifestyle. This could involve stress-reduction methods to boost the immune system and lessen inflammation, such yoga or meditation. Naturopaths may also suggest detoxification regimens to assist in clearing the body of pollutants that may be linked to an excess of yeast.

Through an examination of complementary therapies including acupuncture, homoeopathy, and naturopathy, readers will acquire a more profound comprehension of the possible contribution these therapies can make to the comprehensive therapy of yeast infections. These therapies can complement traditional medical treatments to offer a holistic and individualised approach to healthcare, even though they might not be a complete replacement for them.

It's crucial to remember that not everyone will benefit from alternative therapies, therefore it's crucial to engage with a licenced healthcare provider who can customise a treatment plan for you. Furthermore, since the effects of any alternative therapy may not show up right away, it's imperative to exercise patience and consistency.

Finally, complementary and alternative therapies including naturopathy, homoeopathy, and acupuncture can provide important support for the comprehensive care of yeast infections. These treatments function by correcting the body's underlying imbalances and encouraging self-healing. Readers can equip themselves with extra skills and techniques to manage and prevent yeast infections by investigating these alternative medicines. As always, it's crucial to collaborate with a licenced healthcare provider to create a customised treatment plan that addresses your unique requirements.

# Chapter 4: Customizable Plans for Yeast Infection Management

# Creating a Personalized Treatment Plan

I'll walk you through developing a customised treatment plan in this subchapter to control your yeast infection. We'll take into account things like how serious your infection is, how often it comes back, and your personal preferences. By taking care of these issues, we may create a plan that addresses your lifestyle, beliefs, and general well-being in addition to addressing the underlying cause of your yeast infection.

First, it's critical to recognise that there are differences in the severity of yeast infections. Some people may have modest symptoms that are easily treated, while others may have recurring or chronic infections that seriously decrease their quality of life. We can establish the best course of action and tactics to include in your customised strategy by evaluating the extent of your infection.

Over-the-counter antifungal drugs may be adequate to treat a mild yeast infection, reducing symptoms and curing the illness. These drugs, which come as oral tablets, suppositories, or lotions, function by getting rid of extra yeast and reestablishing the proper balance of vaginal flora. It's crucial to remember that these therapies only offer short-term respite and might not deal with the infection's underlying cause. Therefore, in order to prevent future recurrences and promote general vaginal health, it is imperative to investigate alternative strategies.

A more thorough approach could be required for those with more severe or recurring yeast infections. In these situations, your individualised plan may incorporate antifungal drugs, dietary changes, and additional therapeutic choices. I advise my patients to adopt specific lifestyle changes that can help stop the overgrowth of yeast and create a healthier vaginal environment in addition to taking antifungal drugs.

When it comes to treating yeast infections, diet is very important. Refined carbs and high sugar foods can exacerbate yeast overgrowth, therefore you should minimise your consumption of these foods. Rather, concentrate on eating a well-balanced diet full of foods high in nutrients, like whole grains, fruits, vegetables, lean meats, and healthy fats. Incorporating foods high in probiotics, like kefir, sauerkraut, kimchi, and yoghurt, can also aid in reestablishing the proper balance of vaginal flora.

An extensive treatment regimen should also include regular exercise. Engaging in physical activity promotes vaginal health by increasing blood flow, strengthening the immune system, and assisting with hormone regulation. Exercise on a regular basis can also aid with stress management, as stress is known to impair immunity and raise the risk of yeast infections.

Complementary therapy alternatives can be added to these lifestyle alterations to further improve the efficacy of your customised plan. Garlic, tea tree oil, and coconut oil are examples of natural medicines with antibacterial qualities that can help fight yeast overgrowth. But before utilising these cures, it's crucial to take caution and speak with a healthcare provider because they might not be appropriate for everyone and might trigger allergic reactions or irritation.

Psychological approaches and counselling are very helpful aids in the management of yeast infections. Recurrent or chronic infections can have a negative impact on your mental and emotional health, increasing emotions of annoyance, humiliation, and low self-esteem. You can learn coping mechanisms, manage these feelings, and address any underlying psychological issues that might be causing your infections by working with a counsellor or therapist.

Additionally, your customised approach can include self-help methods like mindfulness exercises, stress management, and relaxation strategies. Stress management and treatment will boost your immune system and lessen the chance of yeast overgrowth.

It is crucial to remember that each person's experience managing a yeast infection is different. Even though the tactics covered in this chapter offer a strong basis, speaking with a healthcare provider is crucial if you want to create a strategy that is customised to your unique requirements. You can express any worries or preferences you may have, look into other treatments, and, as you get well, work with your healthcare practitioner to make any required changes to your plan.

To summarise, developing a customised treatment strategy for managing a yeast infection is essential to treating the underlying causes, avoiding recurrences, and enhancing general vaginal health. Through an evaluation of the extent of your infection, lifestyle changes, integration of supplemental therapies, and psychological considerations, we can create a customised strategy that caters to your individual requirements and preferences. Recall that there is no one-size-fits-all strategy for treating yeast infections; instead, for long-lasting effects, a comprehensive and customised approach is needed.

# Developing Healthy Lifestyle Habits

We explore the role that healthy living practises have in both controlling and preventing yeast infections in this chapter. I have direct experience with the substantial influence that lifestyle decisions may have on our general health and well-being as a medical doctor and health and wellness consultant. Specifically, certain behaviours can be extremely important for managing and preventing yeast infections. This chapter will examine the role that physical activity, good sleep habits, and stress management strategies play in keeping our bodies in a state of balanced health.

Exercise: Moving Towards a Healthier You

Though it goes far beyond that, regular exercise is frequently linked to better cardiovascular health and weight management. Exercise boosts our immune systems in addition to building stronger muscles and increasing our dexterity. Exercise helps flush toxins from the body and promotes the body's natural defences against infections, including yeast infections, by increasing circulation and lymphatic movement.

According to a 2010 University of Illinois study, people who regularly exercised at a moderate to high level were less likely to get recurring yeast infections. Exercise has been demonstrated to promote gut health, lower inflammation, and balance hormone levels—all of which are critical for controlling and avoiding yeast infections.

Aim for at least 30 minutes of moderate-intensity activity most days of the week, such as brisk walking, running, or cycling, to reap the benefits. Including in your programme strength training activities that focus on the main muscle groups might also be advantageous. It's important to start softly and increase the intensity and duration of any new workout regimen gradually.

Sleep Hygiene: Restoring the Body's Natural Balance

In our fast-paced, digitally-savvy world, sleep is frequently neglected. But obtaining enough good sleep is essential for maintaining our general health and wellbeing, which includes managing and preventing yeast infections. Our bodies use sleep as a time for repair and regeneration, which supports healthy hormone balance and a robust immune system.

Our immune systems can be weakened by sleep deprivation, leaving us more vulnerable to diseases, including yeast overgrowth. According to a 2015 study that was published in the journal Sleep Medicine, people who had trouble sleeping had a higher likelihood of getting recurrent yeast infections. In a similar vein, prolonged sleep deprivation has been linked to gut health problems and elevated inflammation, both of which can exacerbate yeast infections.

Developing a regular sleep schedule is essential for bettering sleep hygiene. Aim to go to bed and wake up at the same time every day, and try to get seven or eight hours of unbroken sleep every night. Make sure your bedroom is cold, dark, and clear of distractions like electronics to create a peaceful atmosphere. Better sleep can also be achieved by using relaxation methods before bed, such as mindfulness training or deep breathing exercises.

Stress Reduction Techniques: Finding Inner Balance

Although stress is becoming an unavoidable aspect of modern life, its negative effects on our health should not be overlooked. Prolonged stress may cause havoc on our immune system, throw off hormone balance, and damage our digestive systems, all of which can lead to an overabundance of yeast in the body. The secret to keeping a good balance and avoiding yeast infections is proper stress management.

There are lots of ways to reduce stress that we can apply to our everyday lives. It has been demonstrated that mind-body techniques like yoga, tai chi, and meditation lower stress levels, strengthen the immune system, and increase general wellbeing. By triggering the body's relaxation response, these techniques aid in calming the body and lessening the negative effects of stress.

Taking part in enjoyable and relaxing hobbies or pastimes is another powerful stress-reduction strategy. Finding hobbies that help you relax and remove yourself from daily worries, whether it's painting, gardening, or dancing, can have a significant positive impact on your mental and emotional health.

In addition, having a solid support network is essential for stress management. Look for therapists, family members, or close friends that you can confide in and rely on for assistance when things go tough. Regular check-ins with a health and wellness coach can also offer helpful direction and responsibility regarding stress reduction methods.

In summary, adopting a healthy lifestyle is essential to controlling and avoiding yeast infections. A variety of strategies, including regular exercise, good sleep hygiene, and stress management, can help us keep our bodies in a state of balanced health. By adopting these routines, we may give ourselves the ability to take charge of our health and wellbeing, conquering yeast infections and fostering general vitality. Recall that minor adjustments can result in major gains, so begin by making the initial move toward a healthy you right now!

# Integrating Medical and Holistic Approaches

It's critical to keep in mind that there is no one-size-fits-all treatment for yeast infections. Since every person is different, their treatment strategy should also be customised for them. Medical treatments like antifungal drugs may be useful in reducing symptoms and curing an infection, but they might not get to the bottom of the issue. Here's where adopting a comprehensive approach can pay off.

As a physician and wellness and health coach, I support a multifaceted approach to healthcare. This is taking into account a person's emotional, mental, and spiritual health in addition to the physical components of an illness. We can develop a treatment strategy that takes care of the signs and symptoms of yeast infections as well as their underlying causes by combining medical and holistic methods.

A crucial element of an integrated strategy is a change in lifestyle. In my role as a medical professional, I collaborate closely with my patients to find any lifestyle choices that might be causing them to have yeast infections. This may encompass dietary decisions, personal hygiene routines, stress levels, sleep habits, and additional factors. Through minor yet significant adjustments in these domains, people can significantly lower their chance of recurring illnesses.

When it comes to nutrition, avoiding specific foods that encourage the growth of yeast can be quite beneficial. This includes sugar-rich foods, processed carbs, and alcoholic beverages. Rather, I advise my patients to concentrate on a plant-based, whole-foods diet that is high in nutrients that support the immune system and reduce inflammation. In addition to assisting in the management of yeast overgrowth, this promotes general health and wellbeing.

My treatment regimens typically include a variety of complementary and alternative treatments in addition to dietary modifications. These could consist of aromatherapy, acupuncture, herbal medicines, and more. These methods support the body's harmony and balance in addition to helping to reduce symptoms. We can develop a more long-lasting and sustainable remedy if we treat the body as a whole as opposed to just the infection.

Techniques from psychology and counselling are also crucial parts of an integrated strategy. Yeast infections can be extremely uncomfortable, resulting in both mental and physical distress. Through the provision of counselling and psychological support, we can assist individuals in managing their issues more effectively. This can entail practising relaxation techniques, stress-reduction strategies, and even attending to any underlying traumas or worries that might be exacerbating their illness.

Self-help methods constitute yet another crucial facet of managing yeast infections. I teach my patients several self-care techniques so they can actively participate in their own recovery process. This could involve self-examination, self-care practises, and appropriate hygiene methods. An individual's feeling of well-being and overall result can be considerably enhanced by feeling that they have agency and control over their situation.

Finally, coping mechanisms are essential for controlling and averting yeast infections. I collaborate with my patients to create individualised coping mechanisms that support them in overcoming any obstacles. This could entail mindfulness exercises, stress-reduction strategies, and building a network of supportive family members who can provide advice.

Through the integration of medical and holistic techniques, a comprehensive and well-rounded treatment plan for the management of yeast infections can be developed. This method gives people a better chance of long-term success because it targets the underlying reasons in addition to the symptoms.

To sum up, managing yeast infections can be a difficult and enduring problem. But by adopting a comprehensive strategy that blends medical and other methods, we can provide them a guide for managing yeast infections entirely. We can design a treatment plan that is specific to each patient's needs by taking into account their physical, emotional, mental, and spiritual demands. We can enable people to take charge of their health and well-being by combining dietary adjustments, counselling, alternative and complementary therapies, self-help techniques, and coping mechanisms. By working together, we can get rid of yeast infections and provide the groundwork for long-term, maximum health and vitality.

# Long-Term Maintenance and Prevention

Many who have felt the pain and aggravation of yeast infections frequently consider preventing them from happening again to be of utmost importance. Since I know how depressing the never-ending cycle of recovery and relapse may be, I'm committed to giving you insightful knowledge and practical advice on how to permanently end this pattern.

I've learned from my years of experience as a medical doctor and health and wellness coach that developing a holistic strategy that takes into account a person's entire nutrition, lifestyle, and general state of well-being is the key to long-term prevention. In addition to treating the symptoms, the underlying causes of yeast infections must also be addressed.

Prior to starting this road of long-term care and prevention, it's critical to comprehend the variables that may raise the likelihood of recurring yeast infections. Certain people could naturally have weakened immune systems, which leaves them more vulnerable to diseases. For others, an overabundance of yeast might result from certain lifestyle choices or health issues that upset the delicate balance of microorganisms in the body.

Keeping up a healthy, balanced diet is one of the most crucial long-term maintenance and preventative techniques. Your body can be made less conducive to yeast growth and your immune system can be strengthened by providing it with the proper nutrients. Including probiotic-rich foods like kefir, sauerkraut, and yoghurt can help balance out the good bacteria in your stomach and stop yeast from growing out of control.

In addition, cutting back on sugar and refined carbs is essential to avoiding yeast infections. Since yeast feeds on sugar, you can effectively starve it and slow its growth by consuming fewer sweets, sugary drinks, and processed meals. Rather, concentrate on including plenty of fresh fruits and vegetables, lean proteins, and complete grains in your diet.

It's critical to treat any underlying medical issues that may raise the risk of recurring yeast infections in addition to making dietary adjustments. Diabetes, hormone abnormalities, and compromised immune systems are a few diseases that might exacerbate yeast overgrowth. Through close collaboration with your healthcare team, you can effectively manage these disorders and lower your risk of reinfection.

Long-term maintenance and prevention also greatly benefit from lifestyle adjustments. For example, it's important to avoid using antibiotics excessively because they can upset your body's bacterial balance and encourage yeast overgrowth. If you do need antibiotics, make sure to discuss with your doctor the possibility of taking probiotics at the same time to offset any side effects.

Another crucial element in avoiding yeast infections is keeping up with hygiene. Maintaining a clean and dry genital area is crucial since moisture can foster the growth of yeast. The natural pH balance in the vagina can be upset by strong or scented feminine hygiene products, so when washing, use gentle, unscented soap instead.

In order to promote air circulation and inhibit the accumulation of moisture, it's also a good idea to steer clear of wearing apparel that is too tight and instead choose breathable materials like cotton. Changing out of sweaty training attire or wet swimsuits as soon as possible can also help lower the incidence of yeast infections.

One more essential component of long-term prevention is stress management. Stress can impair immune function and throw off the body's microbial balance, leaving you more vulnerable to illness. Relaxation methods including yoga, meditation, deep breathing, and indulging in enjoyable hobbies can help lower stress levels and enhance general wellbeing.

Last but not least, consistent exercise is crucial for both long-term preservation and prevention. Exercise strengthens the immune system and increases blood circulation, both of which aid in the body's removal of pollutants. On most days of the week, try to get in at least 30 minutes of moderate-intensity activity, such as cycling, dancing, running, or brisk walking.

In conclusion, a thorough strategy that takes into account a person's food, lifestyle, and general health is needed to achieve long-term maintenance and prevention of yeast infections. You may lessen the likelihood of recurrent infections and foster an environment where yeast is less likely to flourish by implementing these techniques into your everyday routine. Always remember that prevention is the key to long-lasting relief and taking back control of your health by using a comprehensive approach.

# Chapter 5: Self-Help Techniques and Coping Strategies

# Emotional Well-being and Yeast Infections

As a physician and health and wellness coach, I have personally witnessed the psychological toll that yeast infections can have on people. Patients frequently express frustration, embarrassment, and sometimes guilt about their conditions to me. As a result, they could have feelings of loneliness and suffer with low self-esteem.

It's critical to acknowledge that yeast infections are more than just medical conditions in order to comprehend their emotional effects. They may have a significant impact on an individual's emotional and mental health. Actually, studies have indicated a link between a persistent yeast infection and elevated levels of stress, anxiety, and depression.

The physical discomfort that yeast infections frequently produce is one factor contributing to this emotional impact. Itching, burning, and discomfort are examples of persistent symptoms that can significantly lower someone's quality of life. These physical symptoms may worsen stress and anxiety levels by causing irritation, difficulty concentrating, and irregular sleep habits.

Yeast infections can cause physical discomfort, but they can also have an impact on a person's self-esteem and body image. Feelings of shame and embarrassment can arise from having a persistent yeast infection, especially if the infection is in a visible region like the mouth or genitalia. This can increase the emotional effects of the infection by causing social disengagement and a reluctance to enter into close connections.

Moreover, treating yeast infections can provide mental difficulties. Many people find it difficult to talk about their symptoms and ask for assistance, which can make the illness worse and increase the psychological damage. Furthermore, the course of treatment itself, which frequently include the use of antifungal drugs and lifestyle modifications, can be debilitating and upsetting. Finding the best course of action may need some trial and error and patience, which can be mentally taxing and discouraging.

In spite of these difficulties, it's critical to understand that people can manage a yeast infection and preserve their emotional health at the same time by using useful tactics.

Above all, it is critical to talk openly about the emotional effects of the infection and to seek help. This can be accomplished by asking a therapist or counsellor for professional assistance, or by confiding in a dependable friend or family member. Speaking about the emotional difficulties can help people find support and affirmation as well as assist them in creating appropriate coping strategies.

Furthermore, self-care routines can be quite important for preserving emotional health. Calming and stress reduction can be achieved by partaking in enjoyable and soothing hobbies like yoga, reading, or taking baths. Prioritizing self-acceptance and self-compassion is also crucial. This acknowledges that yeast infections are a common and treatable ailment and that there is no need for guilt or shame.

To create a successful treatment plan, it's critical to collaborate closely with a healthcare provider. This could entail taking antifungal drugs in addition to dietary and lifestyle adjustments. It could take some time to identify the best course of action, therefore it's critical to be persistent and patient. Monitoring symptoms and determining triggers can also be beneficial, as this can yield important data for continued care.

Addressing any underlying issues that might be causing the yeast infection is also crucial. This may entail assessing lifestyle decisions, such as dietary habits and personal hygiene standards, in addition to recognising and handling stressors. Psychological methods like mindfulness meditation or cognitive behavioural therapy can also help with stress management and anxiety reduction.

Ultimately, it is important to acknowledge and not minimise the emotional toll that yeast infections can have. It is a legitimate and important feature of the illness that has the potential to significantly lower someone's quality of life. Through acknowledging and resolving these emotional obstacles, people can take charge of their health and locate the resources and tactics they require to prosper.

# Building Resilience and Self-Compassion

Maintaining self-care routines and cultivating an optimistic outlook are essential while dealing with yeast infections. It can be difficult to handle the mental and physical difficulties brought on by a yeast infection, but you can go through this process with grace and courage if you develop resilience and self-compassion.

As a physician and health and wellness coach, I have seen firsthand the transformative power of self-compassion and resilience in my patients' recovery. I provide my patients a holistic approach to managing yeast infections, including dietary planning, lifestyle modifications, counselling, and self-care strategies, through my team of professionals from many health and wellness sectors. Combining these techniques increases their ability to bounce back from setbacks, enhances their general health, and gives them the confidence to face yeast infection issues.

Understanding Resilience

The capacity to overcome adversity and adjust to difficult circumstances is known as resilience. It is important to accept stress and suffering as chances for personal development and evolution rather than trying to escape them. Being resilient enables us to meet the difficulties presented by yeast infections head-on without giving up or becoming depressed.

Establishing a support system and giving self-care top priority are crucial for developing resilience. Your resilience can be greatly increased by self-care activities like regular exercise, mindfulness and meditation, and obtaining enough sleep. By nourishing your mind, body, and soul, these activities help you approach the problems caused by yeast infections with a calm and collected attitude.

You can also get the emotional support you need to develop resilience by surrounding yourself with a network of friends, family, and medical experts who understand and validate your experiences. It can also be empowering to share your path with others who have had comparable difficulties since it makes you understand that you are not fighting this battle alone.

Cultivating Self-Compassion

The habit of showing kindness and understanding to oneself, especially when facing challenges, is known as self-compassion. Having a yeast infection can often leave one feeling guilty, ashamed, and responsible for oneself. You can let go of these unpleasant feelings and replace them with love, understanding, and forgiving by practising self-compassion.

It is crucial to have a constructive internal conversation in order to foster self-compassion. When you notice yourself engaging in self-defeating thoughts as a result of your yeast infection, replace them with empowering statements. Remember that your yeast infection does not define you and that you are still deserving of happiness, acceptance, and love.

Taking care of oneself is another effective strategy for developing self-compassion. Make time every day to do the things that make you happy and relax. This can be having a warm bath, engaging in a pastime, giving in to a favourite treat, or spending some quiet time reflecting. Making self-care a priority tells your body and mind that, despite having a yeast infection, you are worthy of love and care.

Developing a Positive Mindset

Keeping an optimistic outlook is crucial for controlling yeast infections. Instead of becoming mired in unfavourable ideas and feelings, it enables you to concentrate on the opportunities for recovery and development. You may change how you feel about yeast infections and look for the positive aspects of the difficulties by changing the way you think about them.

Gratitude is a useful tool for cultivating a positive outlook on life. Every day, set aside some time to think about three things for which you are thankful, no matter how minor or unimportant they may appear. By focusing on the positive aspects of your life rather than the problems, this easy technique helps you develop a positive outlook that promotes resilience and healing.

Visionary techniques are also very effective. Shut your eyes and visualise being liberated from the limitations imposed by a yeast infection. Imagine that you are vibrant, energetic, and in good health. In this visualisation, use all of your senses to experience the warmth of your body, the smells of your surroundings, and the sounds of a happy, healthy life. By putting your ideal result into graphic form, you build a road map for your recovery and cultivate optimism.

Nurturing Self-Care Practices

Taking care of oneself is essential to controlling yeast infections. It includes all of the pursuits and methods that advance your mental, emotional, and physical health. You honour yourself and give your body the love and attention it needs when you make self-care a priority. The following self-care techniques can aid in your recovery process:

1. Follow a yeast infection management plan: Together with your medical team, develop a customised plan that takes into account your unique requirements. This could involve medication, alternative therapy, and dietary changes.

2. Practice good hygiene: To avoid more rashes and pain, keep the afflicted areas dry and clean. Steer clear of abrasive soaps or douches that can upset the delicate balance of your vaginal flora.

3. Choose nourishing foods: Include foods that help maintain a balanced gut flora and a strong immune system. Choose foods high in probiotics, like kimchi, kefir, sauerkraut, and yoghurt.

4. Engage in regular exercise: Engaging in physical activity not only enhances your general health but also strengthens your immune system. Incorporate enjoyable hobbies into your everyday routine, such as yoga, dancing, or walking.

5. Prioritize restful sleep: A healthy sleep schedule is necessary for your body to repair and regenerate. Establish a relaxing bedtime

routine that includes deep breathing exercises, reading a book, or listening to relaxing music.

6. Engage in stress-reducing activities: Prolonged stress can worsen yeast infections and impair your immune system. Seek out stress-relieving and relaxing activities, such mindfulness training, hobbies, or time spent in nature.

You can cultivate an environment that facilitates your body's innate ability to heal and recover from yeast infections by supporting these self-care behaviours.

Conclusion:

Developing self-compassion and resilience are essential for controlling yeast infections. You may overcome yeast infections with grace and courage if you cultivate self-care habits, have a good outlook, and surround yourself with encouraging people.

Recall that the process of healing is one that calls for endurance, self-kindness, and patience. Accept the knowledge and direction provided in this chapter, and use it as a model for managing yeast infections in their entirety.

As long as you use self-compassion and resilience as your compass, you can overcome your yeast infection experience and get back your vibrant health and wellbeing.

# Communication and Support Networks

Throughout the course of my years as a medical professional and health and wellness coach, I have learned how important it is to have support systems and open lines of communication when it comes to treating yeast infections. It is more important to build a network of individuals who can offer emotional support, direction, and understanding along your journey than it is to merely adhere to a treatment plan and take medication.

In order to fully recover from a yeast infection, we must acknowledge that it affects not only our physical health but also our mental and emotional health. People frequently feel ashamed or humiliated by this illness, thinking it's the result of bad personal hygiene or behaviours. I want to reassure you, though, that anyone can get a yeast infection, independent of lifestyle or cleanliness habits. We may dismantle shame-based barriers and show people that they are not the only ones going through this by being open and honest in our conversations about it.

Asking for help from close friends and family members is one of the first stages in creating a solid support system. By discussing your situation with your significant other, family, or close friends, you give them an opportunity to sympathise with you and provide support. Selecting people you can trust and who will react with compassion and understanding is crucial. Recall that talking about your experience shows your strength and resolve in pursuing a healthier lifestyle, not your weakness.

Professionals in the medical field are another essential source of assistance. I have committed my career as a physician to assisting people just like you in overcoming a variety of medical issues, including yeast infections. It is essential to seek medical advice in order to guarantee that you obtain correct information and suitable therapy. It is crucial to be upfront and truthful with a healthcare provider about your symptoms, worries, and any prior therapies you may have tried. By giving them this information, experts can create a treatment plan that is especially suited to your requirements.

Moreover, medical personnel are educated to treat yeast infections on both a physical and mental level. They can offer consolation, information, and direction regarding dietary and lifestyle adjustments, psychiatric counselling, self-care options, self-help methods, and coping mechanisms. With their knowledge, you'll be able to comprehend your illness more fully and discover efficient management techniques.

Apart from family members and medical experts, virtual communities can also serve as a beneficial resource for assistance. Through the internet, people may now connect with others who have gone through similar things, which fosters a sense of understanding and belonging. Online communities offer a forum where you may talk about your worries, pose questions, and get support from others who have experienced similar things. On the other hand, you should be cautious and make sure the information you find online is reliable. Although there are benefits to using online forums, it is crucial to add expert medical advice to the material.

Creating a support network entails more than just asking for help; it also entails expressing your boundaries and wants in an effective manner. It's important to communicate honestly and openly about your symptoms, available treatments, and any difficulties or worries you may be having. You can get the best possible help from others by sharing your experiences. Recall that dialogue is a two-way street. It's equally critical to pay attention to and value the counsel and support that friends, family, medical experts, and online communities have to offer.

Finally, I want to stress how important self-advocacy is. The greatest advocate for your health and wellbeing is ultimately you, even though your support system is crucial. Spend some time learning about yeast infections, their causes, and available treatments. Take the initiative to get the support and assistance you require. Follow your gut and ask inquiries or communicate any concerns you may have. By actively participating in your healthcare, you enhance your quality of life and give yourself the power to make wise decisions.

In summary, creating support networks and having efficient communication are essential parts of controlling yeast infection. Ask for help from family members who are empathetic and have understanding. Speak with medical experts who can offer the required medical direction and psychological assistance. Participate in online forums to meet others who have gone through similar things. Recall to talk honestly and openly while paying attention to the counsel and encouragement that your network has to offer. Above all, make self-advocacy a priority and participate actively in your healthcare process. We can conquer yeast infection and reach our best health and wellbeing together.

# Overcoming Challenges and Celebrating Progress

Managing and recovering from yeast infections is a journey, and there will inevitably be obstacles to overcome. These difficulties could manifest in a number of ways, including medical symptoms, emotional upheaval, and delays in the course of treatment. But it's crucial to keep in mind that obstacles are just chances for development and learning. In order to help you feel empowered and motivated as you work toward mastery over yeast infections, we will discuss methods for conquering these challenges and recognise your accomplishments in this chapter.

1. Acknowledge and Accept the Challenges:

To overcome obstacles, one must first recognise and accept their existence. When faced with setbacks or recurrent symptoms, it is typical to feel overwhelmed, frustrated, or even despair. But it's important to keep in mind that these difficulties don't equal your merit or work. You can change to a more positive and empowered perspective by acknowledging that obstacles are a part of the path.

2. Seek Support and Guidance:

It is never a good idea to travel alone, and treating yeast infections is no different. Seek assistance from medical specialists like me who can offer direction and knowledge specific to your requirements. Making connections with a group of people going through comparable struggles can also be a great way to get support and hear about other people's experiences. You can find comfort in the knowledge that you are not travelling alone by telling and hearing tales of resiliency and victory.

3. Learn from Setbacks and Adjust Your Approach:

Any healing process is inevitably accompanied by setbacks. Consider setbacks as opportunities to grow and learn, rather than as failures. Consider the variables that might have contributed to the setback and pinpoint areas that require modification. This can entail reviewing your treatment regimen, lifestyle decisions, or food. Being proactive and flexible can help you overcome obstacles more skillfully and advance in managing yeast infections more generally.

4. Cultivate Self-Compassion and Patience:

Self-compassion and patience are necessary for managing yeast infections because results aren't always straight-line. It's critical to remember to treat yourself with kindness and accept that recovery takes time. Through all of this journey's ups and downs, practise patience with your body, mind, and emotions. Recall that no matter how minor, your accomplishments should be acknowledged and that defeats do not define you. Developing patience and self-compassion will support you in keeping a good outlook and staying inspired to reach your highest level of wellness.

5. Embrace Holistic Self-Care:

Holistic self-care techniques can significantly accelerate your progress toward mastery over yeast infections in addition to medical treatment. These habits include providing your body with a healthy food, working out frequently, practising mindfulness or relaxation techniques to reduce stress, getting enough sleep, and cultivating wholesome relationships. Making self-care a priority helps you maintain your general health, which helps your body heal and prevents further yeast infections.

6. Set Realistic Goals and Celebrate Milestones:

Establishing attainable objectives and acknowledging accomplishments along the way can provide you a concrete gauge of your development and increase your motivation. Divide your overall plan for managing yeast infections into more manageable, time-bound, detailed, quantifiable, and attainable goals (SMART goals). For instance, you may resolve to reduce your stress levels on a regular basis or increase the amount of foods high in probiotics in your diet. As you accomplish these objectives, give yourself some time to recognise and enjoy your successes. Your sense of empowerment is strengthened by this acknowledgement, which motivates you to keep moving forward with the management of your yeast infection.

7. Practice Mindfulness and Visualization Techniques:

Techniques for visualisation and mindfulness can be very effective in overcoming obstacles and boosting motivation. You can improve your ability to respond to obstacles by cultivating a greater awareness of your thoughts, emotions, and physical sensations via mindfulness practise. Using visualisation techniques, you can picture yourself in an ideal state of health and validate your capacity to overcome obstacles and accomplish your objectives. By rewiring your mentality, these methods can lower anxiety and boost resilience and motivation.

8. Stay Educated and Informed:

Being knowledgeable about yeast infections and how to treat them is essential since "knowledge is power." Learn about the most recent findings, available therapies, and lifestyle choices that can help you on your path. As a member of the medical community, my colleagues and I are committed to giving you accurate and thorough information. You can also increase your knowledge and self-assurance in treating yeast infections by participating in webinars, workshops, or professional consultations.

Recall that failures do not indicate a lack of effort or value on your part while you manage a yeast infection. Accept the trip, ask for help when you need it, and rejoice at every victory. You will cultivate a sense of empowerment and motivation by incorporating these tactics into your life, which will result in a more robust and satisfied approach to mastering yeast infections.

As we go deeper into coping mechanisms, self-help approaches, and complementary and alternative therapies, you can support yourself even more on your path to full control of your yeast infection. Keep reading. By working together, we can provide you with the skills and information need to free yourself from the grip of yeast infections and restore your health and wellbeing.

# Chapter 6: Frequently Asked Questions About Yeast Infections

# Can Yeast Infections Be Prevented?

Preventive Measures:

A multifaceted strategy is needed to avoid yeast infections, which includes changing some aspects of lifestyle and using a few preventive measures. Let's examine these tactics in more detail:

1. Hygiene: Keeping up with hygiene is one of the most crucial preventive strategies. This involves maintaining a clean and dry genital area, particularly after swimming or physical activity. Strong soaps and douches should never be used since they can upset the vagina's natural pH balance and encourage yeast growth. Instead, use mild cleansers and soaps without fragrances.

2. Clothing Choices: Yeast infections can be avoided by dressing loosely and in materials that breathe, like cotton. Clothing that fits too tight might produce a warm, humid atmosphere that is ideal for the growth of yeast. Furthermore, keep in mind that remaining in sweaty clothes or wearing wet bathing suits for extended periods of time can also lead to the development of yeast infections.

3. Sexual Practices: In addition to being vital for preventing STDs, safe sex practises are also essential for preventing yeast infections. Using dental dams or condoms can help lower the chance of transmission by acting as a barrier against yeast. It's crucial to remember that having oral sex might spread yeast infections, thus care should be used when having these private conversations.

4. Antibiotic Use: Although they are necessary to treat bacterial infections, antibiotics can upset the delicate balance of microorganisms in the body, increasing the chance of developing yeast infections. If you are prescribed antibiotics, follow your doctor's instructions and ask about taking probiotics at the same time to help encourage the growth of good bacteria in your body.

Lifestyle Modifications:

Certain lifestyle changes can help lower the risk of yeast infections in addition to preventive measures. You may establish an environment in your body that is less prone to yeast overgrowth by implementing a few easy changes. Let's investigate these changes:

1. Diet: Preventing yeast infections is just one aspect of general wellness that is greatly aided by eating a nutritious diet. Foods heavy in refined carbohydrates and sugar have the ability to encourage the growth of yeast. As a result, it's critical to consume fewer processed and sugary foods. Rather, prioritise a diet that is well-balanced and full of nutritious grains, lean meats, and an abundance of fruits and vegetables. Consuming foods high in probiotics, including yoghurt and fermented veggies, can also aid in fostering a balanced population of beneficial bacteria within your body.

2. Stress Management: Stress has a significant effect on all aspects of our health, including the immune system, which is essential for avoiding yeast infections. It's crucial to include stress-reduction strategies in your everyday routine as a result. This can involve relaxing and joyful activities as well as techniques like yoga, meditation, and deep breathing exercises. You can help your body fight off infections, including yeast infections, by controlling your stress levels.

Risk Reduction Strategies:

Although lifestyle changes and preventive actions can significantly lower the incidence of yeast infections, some people may be more susceptible than others because of underlying factors. It's crucial to use additional risk-reduction techniques in certain situations:

1. Diabetes Management: People who have diabetes have higher blood sugar levels, which puts them at risk for yeast infections. A healthy diet, regular exercise, and medication can help control blood sugar levels and lower the risk of yeast infections in people with diabetes.

2. Hormonal Changes: Yeast infections can become more common during periods of menstruation, pregnancy, or the menopause, among

other hormonal changes. In these situations, you can lower the risk by practising proper hygiene and talking with your healthcare professional about preventive steps.

3. Immune System Support: Yeast infections are more common in people with weakened immune systems, such as those with HIV/AIDS or undergoing cancer therapies. They must collaborate closely with their physician to control their condition and use immune-strengthening techniques to lessen their susceptibility to yeast infections.

You can actively work toward preventing yeast infections by implementing these preventive measures, lifestyle changes, and risk reduction techniques. But it's important to remember that each person is different, and what suits one person might not suit another. It's critical to pay attention to your body, notice any changes or symptoms, and get medical attention when necessary.

Keep in mind that prevention is the key to preserving your best health, and you may have a yeast-free life by being proactive. A look at the many choices for treating yeast infections and the advantages of holistic therapies that address the underlying causes of this ailment will be covered in the upcoming chapter.

# Are Over-the-Counter Treatments Effective?

Before we start, it's important to understand that over-the-counter medications do not treat the underlying causes of yeast infections, even though they can provide momentary respite from their symptoms. A comprehensive approach is necessary to completely eradicate yeast infections, which are caused by an overgrowth of the yeast species Candida, and to prevent future recurrences.

Studies show that antifungal creams available without a prescription, including miconazole or clotrimazole, work well for treating minor cases of yeast infections. These drugs function by going after the Candida fungus, preventing its development, and finally curing the infection. They can be easily applied and used locally because they are usually available as creams, ointments, sprays, or suppositories.

These over-the-counter remedies, when taken as prescribed, can offer prompt relief from burning, itching, and other bothersome symptoms that are frequently connected to yeast infections. It is crucial to remember that these therapies solely deal with the outward signs and symptoms; they do not correct the underlying imbalances that cause yeast infections. As a result, they might not give a long-term remedy, although they might provide momentary relief.

It's also important to recognise that not everyone is a good candidate for over-the-counter remedies. Before using these treatments, certain people should visit a doctor, especially if they are pregnant, have compromised immune systems, have a history of allergies, or are sensitive to antifungal drugs. Moreover, it's critical to see a healthcare provider for additional assessment and direction if symptoms worsen or continue despite taking over-the-counter medications for a few days.

Although over-the-counter medications have the potential to effectively treat moderate cases of yeast infections, they are not a universally applicable cure. It's critical to keep in mind that every person is different and that different people may respond differently to various treatments. Furthermore, it's critical to comprehend the restrictions associated with over-the-counter medications and the circumstances in which consulting a physician may be necessary.

Seeking medical attention is advised if you are suffering from recurrent yeast infections or if your symptoms are severe and long-lasting. To identify the underlying reasons of your yeast infections, a healthcare provider can perform a comprehensive evaluation that may include a detailed medical history, a physical examination, and possibly even laboratory testing.

Effective management and prevention of yeast infections depend on an understanding of their underlying causes. Yeast infections can occasionally be a sign of a more serious medical issue, including diabetes or weakened immune function. You can get rid of the infection right away and lessen the chance that it will come back by treating these underlying causes.

Additionally, a medical expert can provide you individualised treatment suggestions, such as oral probiotics, prescription antifungal drugs, dietary adjustments, and lifestyle changes. These advice are customised to meet your unique needs and address the internal imbalances and exterior symptoms that lead to the development of yeast infections.

It is crucial to handle yeast infections holistically in addition to consulting a medical practitioner. This method entails changing one's way of life, including dietary adjustments, maintaining good hygiene, and forming wholesome routines that enhance one's general wellbeing.

Wearing breathable underwear, staying away from tight clothing, and practising good cleanliness are a few examples of lifestyle adjustments. By taking these steps, you can lessen the growth of yeast in the environment and lower your risk of infection.

Reducing sugar and refined carbohydrate intake is crucial when it comes to nutrition because these can encourage the growth of Candida. Rather, concentrate on including meals high in nutrients, including leafy greens, lean proteins, and foods high in probiotics, like yoghurt and fermented vegetables, which aid in reestablishing the proper balance of good bacteria in your body.

Additionally, using stress-reduction methods like deep breathing exercises, meditation, and regular exercise might boost immunity and lower the risk of yeast infections.

Effective treatment of yeast infections requires knowledge of the limitations of over-the-counter remedies and, when necessary, seeing a physician. You can regulate your health and effectively manage yeast infections by treating interior imbalances as well as the outward symptoms with a comprehensive and holistic approach.

Remind yourself, readers, that you deserve to take time and care for your well-being. Consult medical professionals for advice, change your lifestyle, and take up healthy behaviours to promote your best health. Being knowledgeable and empowered is the first step on your path to total treatment of yeast infections, and I'm here to help you every step of the way.

# How Long Does It Take to Treat a Yeast Infection?

Prior to getting into the specifics, it's critical to realise that because every person's physiology is different, the length of time needed to treat a yeast infection can vary. Nonetheless, we can learn more about the elements that go into the entire therapy plan by comprehending the elements that affect the healing process.

The severity of the infection is one of the main variables that affects how long the treatment for a yeast infection takes. Treatment for mild yeast infections, which are frequently characterised by minimal symptoms like itching and irritation, may usually be completed more quickly. With the right care, these minor instances can usually be resolved in a week or two. Conversely, more serious infections that cause a great deal of swelling, itching, and discharge could take longer to heal. In rare circumstances, total recovery and infection eradication may need several weeks.

The efficacy of the chosen treatment strategy also influences how long a patient will get treatment. Many people with moderate yeast infections turn to over-the-counter antifungal creams and suppositories as their first line of treatment. The suggested treatment period is typically outlined in the instructions that come with these items. Even in cases where symptoms subside before the end of the treatment time, it is imperative that you follow these guidelines and finish the entire course of treatment.

It is strongly advised that you seek expert medical assistance for infections that are more serious or recurrent. For example, oral fluconazole, a tablet form of antifungal medication, might be prescribed by a gynaecologist or healthcare practitioner. These prescription-only drugs are often taken for a longer period of time—between one and three weeks.

But it's important to emphasise that the course of therapy entails not only getting rid of the symptoms but also making sure that any underlying reasons or contributing factors are taken care of. A disruption in the vaginal microbiota, which can be brought on by immune system dysfunction, hormonal fluctuations, or the use of specific drugs, is frequently the cause of yeast infections. In order to stop repeated infections, treating these underlying causes is essential. Therefore, healthcare professionals may advise making extra lifestyle changes and implementing preventive steps in addition to prescribing antifungal medicine.

For instance, controlling and avoiding yeast infections can be greatly aided by dietary modifications. Foods that are heavy in sugar and processed carbohydrates, for example, might encourage the growth of yeast and exacerbate an infection. It may therefore be advantageous to limit the intake of these items in favour of a well-balanced diet that consists of whole grains, lean proteins, healthy fats, and an abundance of fruits and vegetables. Furthermore, consuming probiotic-rich meals or probiotic supplements can assist in maintaining a healthy vaginal microbiota and reestablishing the body's natural balance of bacteria.

Furthermore, treating yeast infections requires adhering to strict hygiene guidelines. This entails changing out of wet or sweaty clothes as quickly as possible, avoiding the use of strong soaps or douches in the genital area, and donning breathable cotton underwear. These actions contribute to the development of an environment that inhibits yeast growth.

Moreover, stress-reduction methods include regular exercise, meditation, and relaxation exercises can help avoid yeast infections. People who experience ongoing stress and have compromised immune systems may be more prone to illnesses. People can boost their immunity and enhance their general health by adopting stress-reduction techniques, which lowers the risk of recurrent yeast infections.

In summary, the length of time needed to treat a yeast infection can vary based on a number of variables, such as the illness's severity, the efficacy of the chosen course of action, and the existence of any underlying causes or contributing factors. If treated properly, mild infections can go away in a week or two, but more serious infections might take several weeks to treat. In order to prevent repeated infections, it is crucial to address any underlying causes or contributing factors and adhere to the specified treatment period, whether using over-the-counter or prescription treatments. Through dietary adjustments, stress reduction methods, and lifestyle changes, people can improve their general well-being and lower their risk of developing yeast infections in the future. Recall that every person's path to effective management of a yeast infection is distinct, and that healing is possible with the right support and care.

# When Should I Consult a Healthcare Professional?

When a yeast infection first appears, it can cause a number of unpleasant symptoms. These symptoms, which can range from burning and itching to vaginal discharge and pain during sexual activity, can have a serious negative effect on a person's quality of life. Even while over-the-counter antifungal creams or suppositories can frequently treat mild symptoms, it's important to know when the infection may need to be treated by a doctor.

Using over-the-counter medicines to ease symptoms but they still persist is one of the most crucial indicators that you should see a doctor. It is imperative that you get medical attention if, after treating your yeast infection for more than seven days, your symptoms have not improved or have gotten worse. If your symptoms are persistent, it's possible that the infection is resistant to regular treatments. In such case, a medical practitioner can prescribe stronger medication to help eradicate the illness more successfully.

The existence of odd or uncommon symptoms is another crucial sign that you should seek medical attention. Itching, burning, and a white discharge like cottage cheese are typical symptoms of yeast infections; however, some signs could point to an underlying illness that needs to be looked into further. For example, it may indicate a more serious infection, such bacterial vaginosis or a sexually transmitted infection, if you have intense discomfort, swelling, or redness in the vaginal area. In situations like these, it's critical to speak with a medical expert in order to rule out any more possible causes and obtain the right therapy.

When a yeast infection is detected in a pregnant woman, it is important to treat it seriously and get help as soon as possible. Due to weakened immune systems, pregnant women are more prone to illnesses. Furthermore, untreated yeast infections during pregnancy might result in difficulties like early labour or a higher chance of giving birth to a child that is underweight. Therefore, in order to protect both the mother's and the unborn child's health and wellbeing, it is imperative that pregnant women seek medical attention as soon as they suspect a yeast infection.

If they suspect a yeast infection, those with weakened immune systems—such as those receiving chemotherapy or living with HIV/AIDS—should also speak with a medical expert. These people are more likely to get infections again or over time, and they might need specific care to get rid of the infection. A healthcare expert will be able to evaluate each person's particular situation and direct them toward the best course of action.

Finally, if this is your first yeast infection or if you have a history of recurring or frequent infections, it is imperative that you see a healthcare provider. First-time infections are occasionally misdiagnosed as sexually transmitted infections or even other vaginal illnesses like bacterial vaginosis. An expert in healthcare will be able to correctly identify the infection and offer you the best course of action. Likewise, people who have a history of repeated yeast infections can benefit from a more extensive assessment because there might be underlying causes of the infections that call for medical attention.

In conclusion, it is critical that people understand the symptoms and indicators of a yeast infection that call for a visit with a medical practitioner. Indications that call for medical attention and intervention include pregnancy, immune system compromise, uncommon or abnormal symptoms, persistent symptoms not alleviated by over-the-counter medication, and new or recurring infections. People can assure the management of their yeast infection and avoid any problems by getting medical attention as soon as possible. Always keep in mind that maintaining your health is a prudent decision that requires consulting a healthcare professional. Your health and well-being are of utmost importance.

# Chapter 7: Practical Tips for Yeast Infection Management

# Maintaining Personal Hygiene

I'll provide you helpful advice on how to manage and avoid yeast infections in this subchapter by focusing on keeping good personal cleanliness. We'll discuss a range of topics, including hygiene, wardrobe selection, and regular bathing practices—all of which are essential for preventing yeast infections.

Let's talk about the significance of appropriate genital care first and foremost. Because the genital area is a delicate area of the body, it needs to be cleaned and kept hygienic on a regular basis to avoid infections. Maintaining cleanliness and dryness of the area is paramount when it comes to genital care. This entails regularly cleaning the vaginal region with warm water and a mild, scent-free soap.

Steer clear of strong soaps and feminine hygiene products that can upset the vagina's natural pH balance since they can foster an environment that encourages the growth of yeast. Additionally, it's critical to keep in mind that wiping after using the restroom should always be done from front to back in order to stop bacteria from moving from the anus to the vagina.

Choosing the right kind of underwear is crucial, in addition to routine cleaning. Select breathable materials, such as cotton, to promote healthy airflow and prevent moisture buildup in the vaginal region. Steer clear of synthetic materials and form-fitting undergarments as they can retain moisture and provide the perfect environment for yeast growth.

Another important step in avoiding yeast infections is to change out of wet clothing as soon as possible, especially swimwear. Extended periods of wetness or moisture can offer the ideal environment for yeast to grow. So, after swimming or any other activity that can create perspiration, make it your routine to change into dry clothes.

Let's now discuss bathing habits. All of us love a good, long, hot bath or shower, but you should pay attention to the temperature and length of your bathing experience. The normal balance of bacteria in the vaginal area can be upset by extreme heat and extended exposure to water, which increases the risk of yeast infections.

Taking brief baths or showers with lukewarm water is advised. Hot water should be avoided as it can deplete the skin of its natural oils, leading to irritation and dryness. Avoid using strong soaps or shower gels that could have chemicals or perfumes that irritate the sensitive skin around the genital area.

Dry the vaginal region carefully with a fresh towel after showering. Rubbing the region firmly can irritate it, so refrain from doing so. Before putting on any clothes or undergarments, make sure the area is totally dry. It is important to always keep the area dry since moisture trapped against the skin provides yeast with the perfect environment to grow.

The development and treatment of yeast infections can be influenced by clothing choices in addition to good genital hygiene and bathing habits. Choose breathable materials, such as cotton, which promotes appropriate air circulation and moisture absorption, as previously discussed. Restrict airflow and create a moist environment that promotes the growth of yeast by avoiding wearing clothing that is too tight, especially in the genital area.

Additionally, it's critical to consider how clean your clothes are. An increased risk of illnesses arises from the harbouring of bacteria and yeast in soiled or dirty underpants. Make sure to use a light detergent to wash your underwear and other personal items on a regular basis. Keep out of the genital area. Harsh chemicals and fabric softeners might hurt the sensitive skin there.

Maintaining personal cleanliness is only one component of the management of yeast infections. It's critical to take a comprehensive strategy that addresses stress reduction, healthy eating, and other lifestyle changes. If you follow these habits on a daily basis, you can lower your chances of getting a yeast infection and treat it successfully if it does.

To sum up, keeping oneself clean is essential to controlling and avoiding yeast infections. The chance of getting a yeast infection can be significantly decreased by according to the useful advice in this subchapter regarding correct genital care, bathing practises, and clothing selection. It is important to maintain proper hygiene practises in your daily routine, select breathable clothing, and keep the genital area dry and clean. Making personal hygiene a top priority is a proactive step toward managing and preventing yeast infections.

# Dietary Guidelines for Yeast Infection Management

Educate yourself about yeast infection-causing foods

You must be aware of the foods that promote the growth and spread of yeast infections in order to treat them properly. Since sugar is what yeast eats, it's critical to consume less sugar and meals that the body breaks down rapidly into sugar. Refined carbs include things like pasta, white bread, white rice, and sugary desserts. It's also a good idea to stay away from packaged and processed foods, as they frequently include added artificial ingredients and hidden sugars.

Focus on anti-inflammatory foods

Including items that are anti-inflammatory in your diet helps boost immunity and lessen inflammation, which is frequently linked to yeast overgrowth. Foods high in omega-3s, such as salmon and sardines, leafy greens, berries, turmeric, and ginger, are examples of anti-inflammatory foods. These foods support general health and wellbeing in addition to being helpful in treating yeast infections.

Include probiotic-rich foods

Probiotics are good bacteria that support a balanced population of germs throughout the body, including the vaginal region. You can lower your risk of yeast infections and help restore the natural balance of bacteria in your body by include foods high in probiotics in your diet. Foods high in probiotics include kombucha, yoghurt, kefir, sauerkraut, and kimchi. Including these foods in your diet can help maintain a healthy gut and vaginal flora by giving your body a consistent supply of good bacteria.

Consider a low-sugar, low-carbohydrate diet

Cutting back on sugar and carbohydrates in general can help you manage yeast infections much better. Foods high in sugar and carbohydrates provide yeast the perfect conditions to grow. You can aid in starving the yeast and stop their overgrowth by implementing a low-sugar, low-carb diet. Rather, concentrate on eating non-starchy vegetables, lean protein, and healthy fats. These foods supply vital nutrients without giving yeast food.

Meal planning tips for yeast infection management

Organizing your meals can help you control yeast infections. You can make sure you always have wholesome, yeast-infection-friendly food on hand by planning your meals in advance. Here are some pointers to get you started with meal planning:

1. Plan your meals around whole, unprocessed foods: This comprises healthful fats, lean proteins, and fresh fruits and vegetables. These foods reduce the chance of yeast overgrowth while supplying vital nutrients.

2. Batch cook and freeze: Make a lot of food that can be quickly frozen and reheated. You'll save time and make sure you always have a nutritious lunch alternative available to you by doing this.

3. Incorporate variety: Try experimenting with different flavours and ingredients without fear. To make your meals interesting and pleasurable, experiment with new dishes and try flavours from other cultures.

4. Pack lunches and snacks: Pack a nutritious snack and lunch for the day so you don't have to rely on processed and sugary meals. By doing this, you can avoid cravings and maintain your diet plan.

Healthy snack options for yeast infection management

Managing yeast infections can make snacking difficult because a lot of popular snack foods are heavy in sugar and carbs. However, you may have tasty and healthful snacks that won't cause yeast overgrowth if you put a little thought and imagination into them. Here are some suggestions to get you going:

1. Fresh vegetable sticks with homemade hummus: Enjoy some sliced carrot, celery, and cucumber sticks with a homemade hummus

dip. Chickpeas, which are an excellent source of fibre and protein, are used to make hummus.

2. Greek yogurt with berries and a sprinkle of cinnamon: Greek yoghurt is a great option for treating yeast infections since it is high in protein and probiotics. Add some taste and antioxidants by topping it with a sprinkling of cinnamon and fresh berries.

3. Avocado and smoked salmon roll-ups: For a tasty and wholesome snack, spread some mashed avocado over a piece of smoked salmon and roll it up. Omega-3 fatty acids, which are abundant in smoked salmon, have anti-inflammatory qualities.

4. Almonds and walnuts: Nuts are an excellent source of protein and good fats. They're a great, portable snack that's easy to eat and digest. Because nuts are high in calories, pay attention to portion amounts.

It's critical to keep in mind that each person has unique nutritional requirements and preferences. One person's solution might not be another's. Before making big dietary changes, it's always a good idea to speak with a medical expert or certified dietitian, particularly if you have any particular health issues or dietary limitations.

You can actively manage yeast infections and enhance general health and well-being by adhering to these dietary recommendations and implementing them into your everyday routine. You may live your life to the fullest and attain optimal health with perseverance, patience, and the correct support.

# Natural Remedies for Symptom Relief

Soothing Techniques:

1. Warm Baths: Taking a warm bath might help reduce inflammation and itching brought on by yeast infections. Another way to stop yeast growth in the bath is to add a few drops of apple cider vinegar or tea tree oil.

2. Ice Packs: Reducing itching and relieving inflammation in the affected area can be achieved by applying an ice pack or cold compress. Apply the ice pack for ten to fifteen minutes at a time, several times a day, after wrapping it in a fresh cloth.

3. Coconut Oil: Because of its antifungal qualities, coconut oil helps reduce inflammation and irritation. Massage a small amount of coconut oil into the afflicted area after applying a thin layer. Do this two or three times a day.

4. Aloe Vera: Aloe vera gel is well renowned for its anti-inflammatory and calming qualities. For prompt pain and itching relief, apply a tiny amount of fresh aloe vera gel to the affected region.

Herbal Remedies:

1. Garlic: As a naturally occurring antifungal, garlic can aid in the destruction of the infected yeast. Using a few crushed garlic cloves, form a paste. After applying the paste to the afflicted area, rinse it off after 30 minutes. Do this two or three times a day.

2. Calendula: Herb calendula is well-known for its antifungal and anti-inflammatory qualities. Calendula oil or cream can be used directly to the afflicted region to reduce inflammation and itching. You may also use a few drops of calendula oil in some warm water to create a calming bath.

3. Tea Tree Oil: Strong antifungal qualities of tea tree oil can aid in the treatment of yeast infections. Apply a small amount of tea tree oil to the affected region by combining it with a carrier oil, like coconut or olive oil. Before washing it off, let it sit for a few hours.

Home Remedies:

1. Yogurt: Probiotics included in yoghurt can aid in reestablishing the proper ratio of beneficial bacteria in the body, preventing the overabundance of yeast. On the afflicted region, apply plain, unsweetened yoghurt. Let it sit for a few hours before rinsing it off. Yogurt is another food you may eat every day to support intestinal health in general.

2. Apple Cider Vinegar: Apple cider vinegar can aid in the removal of yeast due to its antifungal and antibacterial qualities. Use a combination of equal parts apple cider vinegar and water as a rinse or douche. Repeat one or two times daily until the symptoms subside.

3. Cranberry Juice: Although it can also help with yeast infections, cranberry juice has long been used to treat and prevent urinary tract infections. Sip pure, unsweetened cranberry juice to help relieve symptoms and remove yeast from your body.

To stop yeast infections from returning, it's crucial to follow certain lifestyle guidelines and practise proper cleanliness in addition to using these natural treatments. Practicing basic hygiene, avoiding clothing that is too tight, and wearing breathable cotton underwear can all help prevent yeast infections.

Always remember that even while natural cures have their advantages, you should always speak with a doctor before beginning any new treatment regimen, particularly if you are pregnant or have underlying medical concerns. Your physician can offer you individualised advice and guarantee that the treatments are both safe and efficient for you.

In summary, treating yeast infections requires both treating the underlying cause and reducing their irritating symptoms. Incorporating home remedies, herbal cures, and soothing techniques into your treatment plan will help you heal naturally and holistically while also efficiently relieving discomfort.

# Incorporating Self-Care Practices

As a physician and health and wellness coach, I have seen firsthand how self-care routines can significantly improve the lives of my patients. I've witnessed people who have battled recurring yeast infections find relief and regain control over their health by implementing stress-reduction tactics, relaxation methods, and self-care routines.

Prior to delving further into this subject, let us clarify what self-care actually entails. Fundamentally, self-care is the intentional decisions and acts we take to promote our mental, emotional, and physical well. It entails accepting accountability for our health and making choices every day that promote our general well-being.

It becomes even more important to exercise self-care when it comes to controlling yeast infections. These procedures attempt to treat the infection's underlying causes in addition to relieving its symptoms. Your everyday routine can establish a solid basis for long-term health and well-being by including self-care.

Finding self-care routines that you enjoy is one of the first stages towards implementing self-care practises. When it comes to self-care, everyone has different needs and interests, so it's important to try out different hobbies to see which one speaks to you specifically.

Taking a warm bath with Epsom salts, essential oils, or calming herbs like chamomile might provide comfort to certain people. Taking some time for yourself to relax and soak in the healing powers of water can help reduce the symptoms of yeast infections and promote physical relaxation.

Others might find comfort in doing focused meditation or light yoga. Engaging in these sports fosters not just physical strength and flexibility but also mental clarity and inner serenity. Particularly, yoga has been demonstrated to improve immune system performance, hormonal balance, and stress reduction—all of which might have an impact on the management of yeast infections.

Relaxation techniques are an essential component of self-care routines. Prolonged stress can have disastrous effects on the body, impairing immunity, upsetting hormonal balance, and increasing the risk of yeast infections. You may effectively lower your stress levels and strengthen your body's natural defences against infections by learning and implementing relaxation techniques.

Deep breathing is one such method. Taking slow, deep breaths allows the diaphragm to expand and properly oxygenate the body. This is a simple technique. It has been demonstrated that deep breathing activates the parasympathetic nervous system, which lessens stress and encourages relaxation.

Another useful method is progressive muscle relaxation, which is methodically tensing and relaxing various bodily muscular groups. This exercise develops a deeper sense of peace and relaxation in addition to assisting with physical tension release.

Techniques for reducing stress are also crucial for managing yeast infections. The immediate effects of stress on the body can be addressed by self-care routines and relaxation techniques, but preventing repeated yeast infections may also depend on recognising and addressing stressors in your life.

Examine your daily schedule and note any places where tension seems to be building up. Are there any obligations—personal or professional—that are too great and putting you under unnecessary stress? Are there any emotionally taxing relationships in your life? Once you've identified these stressors, you may start formulating plans to lessen their negative effects on your health.

For instance, you might think about putting time management strategies into practise, establishing boundaries, and engaging in productive stress communication with coworkers or superiors if work-related stress is a major concern. Seeking professional assistance or participating in therapy may offer insightful information and helpful coping mechanisms if relationships are a source of stress.

Getting into a regular workout programme is another effective stress-reduction method. Exercise releases endorphins, which are the body's natural compounds that elevate mood in addition to improving physical health. Whether it's doing yoga, taking brisk walks, or playing your favourite sport, choosing an activity you enjoy can make a big difference in your general wellbeing and stress reduction.

Finally, for long-term success, self-care habits must be a part of your plan for managing yeast infections. You can develop a comprehensive strategy for treating your yeast infections by learning self-care routines, embracing relaxation techniques, and putting stress management tactics into practise.

Recall that taking care of oneself is essential, not optional. Put your health first and make deliberate decisions every day to maintain it. Self-care is the first step in managing a yeast infection completely, and if you follow this path, I guarantee that your health and general well-being will improve dramatically.

# Chapter 8: Navigating Intimate Relationships With Yeast Infections

# Communicating With Your Partner

1. Choose the right time and place:

The right time and place are crucial for establishing a fruitful discussion when talking about any sensitive subject. Select a moment when both of you are at ease and have enough privacy to have a candid conversation. It may be a nice stroll outside or a laid-back evening at home. Establishing a welcoming environment will promote candid dialogue and lessen any possible feelings of guilt or humiliation.

2. Educate yourself:

Learn as much as you can about yeast infections before talking about them with your significant other. Recognize the causes, signs, available treatments, and preventative measures. You will be better able to reassure and encourage your spouse and respond to any queries they may have if you are well-versed in the subject.

3. Use non-judgmental language:

It is imperative that you approach the discussion with compassion and comprehension. It will be easier to provide a safe space for your spouse to voice their concerns and ask questions if you speak without passing judgement. Steer clear of criticism and blame and concentrate on how crucial it is to collaborate in order to effectively treat the illness.

4. Explain the causes and symptoms:

Numerous conditions, such as immunocompromised patients, hormonal fluctuations, and certain drugs, can result in yeast infections. Talk to your spouse about these reasons and the typical symptoms, which include burning, itching, and vaginal discharge. You may help your spouse understand the physical impacts you are going through and how it might affect your closeness by sharing this information with them.

5. Address misconceptions and concerns:

There are a few common myths about yeast infections that may cause uncertainty or unwarranted anxiety. Seize the chance to clear up any misunderstandings your spouse might have and give truthful facts. For instance, make it clear that infidelity or poor cleanliness do not cause yeast infections. You can allay your partner's worries by giving them concise, accurate explanations.

6. Encourage open dialogue and questions:

Invite your companion to share any worries they may have and to ask questions. Let them express their ideas and emotions, and listen to them without interjecting. Always keep in mind that encouraging understanding and support requires open communication. Use your medical knowledge to successfully address any concerns while exercising patience and giving honest answers.

7. Discuss treatment options:

Prescription or over-the-counter drugs are useful treatments for yeast infections. Give your partner this information and go over the various available treatment options. Talk about any potential risks or safety measures, and stress how crucial it is to follow the prescribed course of action. If need, include your spouse in your regimen, making sure they comprehend the importance of taking medication as directed.

8. Emphasize preventive measures:

An important part of treating yeast infections is prevention. Talk to your partner about preventive steps including avoiding allergens, donning cotton underwear that breathes, and practising proper personal hygiene. Stress the value of healthy living, stress reduction, and appropriate diet in preventing repeated infections. You can collaborate with your spouse to reduce the chance of recurrent infections by including them in these conversations.

9. Seek emotional support:

Managing a yeast infection can pose emotional difficulties, so having your partner's support is essential. Tell them about your feelings and worries, and how the virus has affected your general health. Talk about the various coping mechanisms that can be employed, such as mindfulness exercises, relaxation techniques, and, if necessary, obtaining professional assistance. Encourage your spouse to act as your emotional compass at this time, giving you the understanding and assistance you require.

10. Maintain intimacy:

Intimacy in a relationship can occasionally be impacted by a yeast infection. Talk about any worries or discomfort you may be experiencing with sexual activity, and look into other options for keeping intimacy throughout this time. Make sure that both partners are at ease and respected at all times, and be transparent about any restrictions or safety measures that must be followed.

Recall that communication is an ongoing endeavour. Maintain contact with your partner and bring up the subject again if needed. Motivate them to take an active role in helping you manage your yeast infections since their understanding and support can have a big impact on your overall health.

To sum up, having a successful communication style is essential when talking to your partner about yeast infections. You can promote understanding, empathy, and mutual support by selecting the appropriate time and location, speaking in a nonjudgmental manner, educating yourself and your partner, clearing up any misunderstandings and worries, promoting an open dialogue, talking about treatment options and preventive measures, asking for emotional support, and preserving intimacy. Working together, you may overcome the difficulties caused by yeast infections and improve your relationship by having honest and polite conversations.

# Safe Sexual Practices and Yeast Infections

As a physician and health and wellness advisor, I am aware of the significance of safe sexual behaviour in halting the spread and recurrence of yeast infections. I will walk you through the several approaches you may take to limit the danger of yeast infections and maintain sexual health in this chapter. You can have a satisfying sexual life without worrying about repeated infections if you include these methods into your routine.

The Use of Barrier Methods

1.1 Condoms: Using condoms is one of the easiest and best ways to safeguard yourself against STDs, including yeast infections. Condoms not only establish a physical barrier between spouses but also stop bodily fluids from being exchanged that can harbour microbes that cause yeast. For optimal protection, condom use must be consistent and appropriate.

1.2 Dental Dams: Dental dams are a great option for people who have oral-genital contact since they lower the incidence of yeast infections. Dental dams are tiny sheets that serve as a barrier between the genitalia and the mouth. They are composed of latex or polyurethane. You can enjoy oral sex while reducing the risk of contracting or spreading a yeast infection by wearing dental dams.

1.3 Gloves: Wearing gloves might give an extra degree of protection if you do manual stimulation or penetration. Since latex and nitrile gloves are less likely to trigger allergic responses, they are advised. You can lower the risk of infection transmission by wearing gloves to protect your hands from any direct contact with organisms that cause yeast infections.

Maintaining Sexual Health

2.1 Personal Hygiene: Maintaining proper personal hygiene is essential for avoiding yeast infections. Washing the genital area carefully with warm water and mild, unscented soap is crucial. Steer clear of strong soaps, douches, and perfumed items since these may upset the vagina's normal bacterial and yeast balance. Furthermore, it's critical to completely dry the vaginal area after washing or showering to avoid moisture accumulation, which might promote yeast overgrowth.

2.2 Urinating Before and After Sexual Activity: Flush away any bacteria or yeast that may have entered the urinary tract before and after sexual activity. Urinary tract infections frequently occur with yeast infections; one easy step can lower your risk of getting both. You can reduce the likelihood of bacterial or yeast overgrowth in the urinary tract, which can result in illness, by emptying your bladder.

2.3 Limiting the Use of Antibiotics: Antibiotics are essential for treating bacterial infections, but they can also upset the body's normal bacterial and yeast balance. Antibiotic use that is prolonged or frequent can encourage the growth of yeast, which can result in infections. It's critical to avoid overusing antibiotics and look into other forms of treatment wherever feasible. Speak with your healthcare provider about ways to reduce the risk of yeast overgrowth if you do need to take antibiotics.

Communication and Shared Responsibility

3.1 Open Communication: Maintaining sexual health requires you and your partner to have open and honest conversation. Talk to your partner about any past yeast infections you may have had and educate them on the illness. If they encounter any symptoms, urge them to get medical advice and treatment. Together, you can stop the spread and recurrence of yeast infections by exchanging this knowledge.

3.2 Mutual Responsibility: It's a joint obligation between spouses to maintain sexual health. It is imperative that both parties take proactive measures to stop the spread of yeast infections. It's critical to support your partner in using barrier techniques regularly, keeping themselves clean, and getting help if needed. You may establish a mutually beneficial and healthy sexual atmosphere by cooperating.

Conclusion:

You may reduce your risk of developing yeast infections and have a satisfying, worry-free sexual life by practising safe sexual behaviour and taking care of your sexual health. Always remember to maintain proper personal cleanliness, communicate honestly with your partner, and apply barrier techniques on a regular basis. You are actively improving your general health and lowering your risk of recurring illnesses by following these instructions. Remain vigilant, educated, and in charge of your sexual well-being.

# Intimacy and Emotional Connection

Many people may have feelings of embarrassment or self-consciousness when they have a yeast infection, which might lower their desire for closeness. It's important to keep in mind that having a yeast infection does not make you less desirable or valuable as a mate. Keeping the lines of communication open with your partner about your emotions, worries, and fears is essential to preserving closeness.

Investigating non-sexual kinds of connection is one of the most important ways to manage a yeast infection without sacrificing intimacy. This can entail doing things together, like holding hands, snuggling, or massaging one another, that promote emotional intimacy. While your body heals, you can continue to strengthen your emotional connection with your partner by concentrating on non-sexual expressions of affection.

In any relationship, communication is key, especially when discussing the difficulties of managing a yeast infection. It's critical to discuss your symptoms, treatment strategy, and any worries you may have with your partner. Not only can an honest and open discussion help allay any fears or anxieties, but it also strengthen your emotional bond.

It is recommended that both couples become knowledgeable about yeast infections. You can address the situation with knowledge and empathy if you are aware of the causes, symptoms, and available treatments. As you collaborate to control the virus, this information you have in common will make your relationship stronger.

Yeast infections occasionally cause emotions of loneliness or annoyance. Acknowledging and validating these feelings is crucial for both you and your relationship. You can strengthen your emotional bond and provide a safe environment for emotional expression by having honest, nonjudgmental talks with others about your experiences.

Developing self-care routines can also improve your intimacy and emotional health. Taking care of yourself, enjoying enjoyable hobbies, and making self-care a priority can help you feel more confident and at ease with who you are. Intimacy and emotional connection with your partner are easier to sustain when you feel good about yourself.

You should prioritise non-sexual intimacy, honest communication, and self-care at this period, but you should also be aware of your partner's needs. One way to help children feel supported and connected is to routinely check in with them, ask about their feelings and concerns, and attend to their needs. Recall that intimacy is a two-way street and that both couples must put forth effort to sustain an emotional connection.

It could be beneficial for certain people to look for professional counselling or treatment. A therapist can offer direction and encouragement, assisting you in overcoming the psychological obstacles associated with treating a yeast infection. They can also offer resources for preserving closeness and emotional connection as well as support candid communication.

Ultimately, it's critical to be patient with the healing process and to have reasonable expectations. It takes time to treat a yeast infection, so it's critical to give yourself time to heal both physically and psychologically. Through empathy, tolerance, and encouragement, you can fortify your emotional bond and emerge from this experience with a stronger one.

In summary, maintaining closeness and emotional connection in your relationship does not have to be sacrificed in order to treat a yeast infection. Yeast infections can be managed while maintaining and fostering your emotional bond by putting tactics like non-sexual intimacy, open communication, self-care, and getting professional help into practise. Remind yourself that you are not travelling alone and that you and your companion are capable of overcoming whatever challenges you may face with tolerance, compassion, and love.

# Seeking Professional Support for Couples

For couples struggling to overcome the difficulties caused by yeast infections, couples therapy is a very helpful resource. It offers a secure environment for both couples to communicate their worries, anxieties, and annoyances. Couples can learn stress-reduction tactics, efficient communication approaches, and relationship-building exercises in therapy. Additionally, therapy can assist in addressing the psychological effects—such as feelings of guilt, embarrassment, or shame—that yeast infections may have on both partners.

Studies have indicated that couples who attend therapy report feeling more satisfied with their relationship and having better communication skills. In comparison to couples who did not seek professional assistance, couples who engaged in treatment reported better levels of relationship satisfaction, according to a study published in the Journal of Marital and Family Therapy. The study also discovered that couples therapy significantly enhanced the quality of relationships overall and improved communication styles and conflict resolution techniques.

Another helpful resource for couples with yeast infections is sexual counselling. These infections can cause pain, discomfort, and a decrease in desire, which can have a major effect on sexual intimacy. Couples can examine their difficulties and come up with solutions that work for both of them in a secure and accepting environment that is provided by sexual counselling.

In a study that was published in the Journal of Sexual Medicine, researchers discovered that women with recurrent vulvovaginal candidiasis (RVVC), a common form of yeast infection, had considerably better sexual function after receiving sexual counselling. The main topics of discussion in the counselling sessions included methods for addressing sexual difficulties, personalised treatment plans, and information regarding the virus. The participants' general quality of life improved, their sexual satisfaction increased, and their symptoms significantly decreased as a result of receiving sexual counselling, according to the findings.

Couples impacted by yeast infections might benefit greatly from the emotional support and affirmation that support groups can offer. By joining a support group, people can meet people going through similar things, exchange stories, and get insightful advice and coping mechanisms. These organisations can be a source of inspiration and encouragement as well as a feeling of community and belonging.

In a study that was published in The Journal of Sexual Medicine, researchers discovered that vulvovaginal candidiasis patients' psychological wellbeing improved when they joined a support group. The study participants said they felt more empowered and in control of their illness, and they felt less alone in their experience. Furthermore, the support group gave people a forum to share helpful pointers and counsel, which improved their capacity to effectively treat their yeast infections.

In my work, I have seen firsthand the life-changing potential of expert assistance for partners battling yeast infections. Benefits from the virus go beyond its physical manifestations and significantly influence these people's emotional health and interpersonal dynamics.

Seeking expert assistance increases the likelihood of better intimacy, communication, and teamwork among partners coping with the difficulties caused by yeast infections. They get knowledge on how to deal with the ups and downs of the infection, find comfort in the experiences that others have had, and get a better comprehension of one another's needs and worries.

It is crucial to remember that asking for professional help shows a dedication to one's relationship and personal well-being rather than weakness or failure. Recognizing how yeast infections affect one's life and seeking advice from qualified experts who can offer the required resources and assistance requires bravery.

I advise couples who are experiencing yeast infections to think about the advantages of support groups, couples therapy, and sexual counselling. These materials can play a crucial role in easing emotional strain and assisting people in creating useful coping mechanisms. Couples can overcome the difficulties caused by yeast infections and succeed in their quest for total yeast infection management by placing a high priority on their emotional and interpersonal well-being.

I will offer helpful hints and recommendations for locating the appropriate experts, resources, and support systems in the upcoming chapters. By working together, we can enable couples to successfully negotiate the challenges posed by yeast infections and create a happy, healthy, and successful partnership.

# Chapter 9: Yeast Infections and Pregnancy

# Yeast Infections and Pregnancy: What You Need to Know

The proliferation of the fungus Candida in the body is the cause of yeast infections, sometimes referred to as candidiasis. Although they can happen anywhere on the body, including the mouth, throat, and skin, yeast infections are most frequently linked to the genital area. Candida albicans, a type of fungus that naturally exists in the body but can cause an imbalance when it grows excessively, is the main cause of these infections.

Hormonal changes in the body during pregnancy can provide the perfect conditions for Candida to overgrow. Particularly, the spike in oestrogen levels might upset the normal microbial balance in the vaginal region, increasing the risk of yeast infections. Infections and the growth of Candida can also be facilitated by the elevated amounts of glycogen, a type of sugar, in vaginal secretions during pregnancy.

Risks:

Although yeast infections are typically not thought to be dangerous during pregnancy, if ignored, they can nonetheless be uncomfortable and provide some hazards. The signs and symptoms of a pregnancy-related yeast infection are comparable to those of a non-pregnant person and can include burning, itching, pain, and unusual discharge. On the other hand, pregnant women can be more vulnerable to recurring infections, which could worsen their discomfort and have an adverse effect on their general health.

Untreated yeast infections may occasionally result in pregnancy-related issues. For example, pelvic inflammatory disease (PID), which can result in infertility or an ectopic pregnancy, can be brought on by an infection that travels to the uterus or fallopian tubes. Furthermore, there is a slim chance that the infant will have a diaper rash from the fungal overgrowth or an oral yeast infection known as thrush if the infection is present during labour and delivery.

Treatment Options:

Pregnancy-related yeast infections must be managed, and this requires careful consideration of the safety and effectiveness of available treatments. As a holistic medical professional, I always give preference to all-natural, non-invasive methods. On the other hand, there are some situations in which the development of the unborn child as well as the health of the pregnant woman may require conventional medical interventions.

Antifungal drugs, usually in the form of vaginally injected creams or suppositories, are part of the conventional treatment for yeast infections. These drugs function by focusing on Candida overgrowth and reestablishing the proper balance of bacteria in the vaginal region. Even while taking these drugs while pregnant is generally safe, it's still advisable to speak with your doctor before beginning any therapy.

Pregnancy-related yeast infections can be treated with a variety of natural treatments and lifestyle changes in addition to medicine. These consist of:

1. Probiotics: Yogurt, kefir, and sauerkraut are examples of foods high in probiotics that you can include in your diet to assist your body's natural microbiome balance be restored. Beneficial bacteria included in probiotics have the ability to control Candida growth and enhance a strong immune system.

2. Hygiene practices: Keeping the genital area clean is crucial to controlling and avoiding yeast infections. Douching should be avoided since it might upset the delicate balance of germs and raise the danger of illness. Instead, use water and mild, fragrance-free soap to gently clean.

3. Cotton underwear: The risk of yeast infections can be decreased by wearing loose-fitting underwear made of breathable fabrics, such cotton, which can help prevent excessive moisture and improve airflow.

Steer clear of synthetic or tight-fitting undergarments as they might retain moisture and foster an environment that is conducive to the establishment of Candida.

4. Balanced diet: A healthy immune system is essential for preventing and treating yeast infections, and it is mostly maintained by a well-balanced diet. Make an effort to include whole foods in your meals, such as fruits, vegetables, whole grains, lean meats, and healthy fats. Reduce the amount of processed foods and refined sugars you consume because these can exacerbate Candida overgrowth.

Preventive Measures:

Preventive care can greatly lower the chance of developing yeast infections during pregnancy. Here are some pointers to remember:

1. Practice good hygiene: Regularly wash the genital area with a light soap and water, and be sure to completely dry it afterwards to avoid leaving any moisture behind.

2. Avoid irritants: Avoid scented hygiene products, bubble baths, and fragrant soaps since these might upset the normal balance of germs in the vaginal region.

3. Wear breathable clothing: To provide adequate ventilation and reduce the accumulation of moisture, choose clothing that fits loosely and is composed of natural materials like cotton.

4. Change wet clothing promptly: To stop yeast growth, change out of wet clothes as soon as you can after working out or swimming.

5. Avoid unnecessary antibiotics: Antibiotics can upset the body's bacterial equilibrium, even if they could be required in specific situations. Antibiotics should only be taken as directed by your doctor.

Conclusion:

If left untreated, yeast infections during pregnancy can be uncomfortable and even dangerous. Nonetheless, they can be successfully controlled and avoided with the appropriate information and preventative actions. Pregnant women can lessen the effect of yeast infections on their general health by being aware of the possible risks, investigating treatment options, and taking preventive steps. As usual, it is crucial to speak with your healthcare practitioner to guarantee that you receive individualised attention and direction during your pregnancy.

# Safe Treatment Options for Pregnant Individuals

The excess of the fungus Candida is the cause of yeast infections, sometimes referred to as vaginal candidiasis. Symptoms like burning, itching, and a thick, white discharge may result from this. Hormonal changes during pregnancy can disrupt the vagina's bacterial and yeast balance, raising the risk of yeast infections. Yeast infections must be treated right once in order to reduce discomfort and avoid any problems.

It is essential to speak with your healthcare physician before beginning any medication or treatment for yeast infections during pregnancy. They will be able to evaluate your particular situation and choose the best course of action for you. Nonetheless, there are a number of safe therapy choices that are frequently suggested for expectant mothers.

During pregnancy, topical creams are frequently the first line of treatment for yeast infections. Antifungal drugs found in these creams may aid in the removal of the infection and the reduction of symptoms. Miconazole and clotrimazole are a couple of the often utilised topical treatments. These drugs function by either eliminating the fungus or stopping its development. When using these lotions, it's crucial to adhere to the directions on the container or those given by your doctor.

Another safe and efficient treatment for yeast infections during pregnancy is suppositories. To treat the infection, they are placed into the vagina and release medicine. Boric acid is one suppository that is frequently utilised. Because of its antifungal qualities and ability to balance the vagina's pH levels, boric acid can help make the environment less conducive to yeast growth. It is significant to remember that using boric acid suppositories incorrectly can result in difficulties and should only be done under a doctor's supervision.

Many pregnant women look for natural treatments to treat yeast infections in addition to traditional ones. It's crucial to keep in mind that, even while natural remedies could be relieving, they should never be used in place of appropriate medical care; rather, they should always be used in addition to medical counsel.

Yogurt is one natural treatment that is deemed safe for use by expectant mothers. Lactobacillus acidophilus, a type of beneficial bacteria found in yoghurt, can aid in restoring the proper balance of vaginal flora and preventing the overabundance of yeast. Itching and pain can be relieved by applying plain, unsweetened yoghurt to the afflicted area or by putting a tampon soaked in yoghurt within the vagina.

Tea tree oil is an additional natural medicine that has been utilised for ages. Yeast infections may be fought off by the antifungal and antibacterial qualities of tea tree oil. But before applying tea tree oil to the affected region, it must be diluted with a carrier oil, like coconut oil. Pregnant women should not use undiluted tea tree oil since it can irritate their developing foetus.

An additional all-natural treatment for yeast infections is garlic. Allicin, a substance found in garlic, has antifungal effects. Putting a clove of garlic in the vagina overnight can help reduce discomfort and fight yeast buildup. It's crucial to remember that this medication should only be taken sparingly because it irritates certain people.

It's vital to keep in mind that while these natural cures could offer comfort, their efficacy might not match that of more traditional therapies. It is advisable to speak with your healthcare physician before beginning any natural pregnancy therapies.

Pregnant women can take preventative measures to avoid developing or reoccurring yeast infections in addition to these treatment choices. Keeping up with basic hygiene, which includes avoiding the use of douches and perfumed items and dressing in breathable cotton underwear, will help stop the overgrowth of yeast. To promote general vaginal health, it's also critical to control stress, eat a balanced diet, and lead a healthy lifestyle.

Finally, it should be noted that having yeast infections during pregnancy can be upsetting and uncomfortable. To help manage and lessen symptoms, safe and efficient therapy alternatives are offered. Itching and pain can be relieved with topical creams, suppositories, and natural therapies like yoghurt, tea tree oil, and garlic. For the best results, it is crucial to discuss any proposed course of action with your healthcare professional before beginning it and to heed their advice. Pregnant women can effectively manage yeast infections and concentrate on enjoying the path to motherhood by being proactive in preventing yeast infections and receiving treatment in a timely manner.

# Preventive Measures and Lifestyle Modifications

Hygiene Practices:

Especially during pregnancy when one is more vulnerable to such illnesses due to hormonal changes, hygiene is crucial in preventing yeast infections. In order to keep the vaginal area clean and clear of any dangerous bacteria or fungi, it's critical to practise good hygiene. The following are some hygiene guidelines that expectant mothers should adhere to:

1. Regularly washing the genital area: It's crucial to maintain cleanliness in the vaginal region to stop yeast overgrowth. Wash the area carefully with a gentle soap that doesn't smell. Steer clear of strong-smelling creams and soaps as they might upset the vagina's natural pH balance and raise the risk of infection.

2. Wiping from front to back: Whether or not you are pregnant, you should all adhere to this fundamental hygiene protocol. Always wipe from front to back when using the restroom to avoid transferring bacteria from the anal to the vaginal region.

3. Avoiding douching: Douching throws off the vaginal area's normal microbial and fungal balance, increasing the risk of yeast infections. During pregnancy, it's advisable to stay away from douching completely and to wash your hands frequently with water and a light soap.

Diet:

Our general health and welfare are greatly influenced by the food we eat. Furthermore, a healthy, well-balanced diet can have a big impact in preventing yeast infections. Pregnant women can lower their risk of yeast infections by implementing the following dietary changes:

1. Reducing sugar intake: Since yeast thrives on sugar, it's critical to consume fewer sugar-containing foods and drinks. Desserts, sodas,

fruit juices, and refined sweets all fall under this category. Rather, concentrate on eating entire, low-sugar fruits like pears, apples, and berries.

2. Incorporating probiotics: Probiotics are good bacteria that support the preservation of a balanced population of germs throughout the body, including the vagina. Preventing yeast infections during pregnancy can be achieved by including foods high in probiotics in your diet. Fermented foods including kefir, sauerkraut, kimchi, and yoghurt are great sources of probiotics.

3. Adding garlic and cranberries: It has been shown that cranberries and garlic both have antifungal qualities that can aid in the prevention of yeast infections. Add garlic to your food or take supplements containing garlic, and think about drinking cranberry juice or adding dried cranberries to your diet.

Overall Wellness:

A healthy lifestyle is essential for avoiding yeast infections during pregnancy, in addition to following proper hygiene procedures and making dietary changes. Pregnant women can alter their lifestyle in the following ways to enhance their general health and lower their risk of yeast infections:

1. Managing stress levels: Stress during pregnancy can have a negative impact on one's immune system, increasing susceptibility to illnesses. Stress-relieving practises like yoga, meditation, deep breathing exercises, and other relaxation methods can lower the incidence of yeast infections and help maintain a healthy immune system.

2. Wearing breathable clothing: Particularly if made of synthetic materials, tight clothing has the potential to retain heat and moisture, which can foster the growth of yeast. Choose airy, loose-fitting clothes composed of natural fibres like cotton to promote healthy airflow and lower your chance of developing yeast infections.

3. Avoiding unnecessary antibiotic use: Antibiotics raise the risk of yeast infections and can upset the normal balance of germs in the

body, including the vagina. When expecting, it's crucial to refrain from taking antibiotics for an extended period of time unless a doctor has prescribed them.

4. Practicing safe sex: It is possible to lower the risk of STDs, which raises the possibility of yeast infections, by practising safe sexual behaviour. The use of barrier techniques, like condoms, can boost defences and stop the spread of dangerous fungus or germs.

It's crucial to remember that although these lifestyle changes and preventative steps can dramatically lower the chance of yeast infections, complete immunity may not be guaranteed. You should see a doctor for a correct diagnosis and treatment if you think you may have a yeast infection or if your symptoms don't go away after trying these remedies.

In conclusion, the best ways to lower the risk of yeast infections during pregnancy are through lifestyle changes and preventative measures. Pregnant women can drastically reduce their risk of acquiring a yeast infection by practising good hygiene, changing their diet, and emphasising general wellbeing. During this wonderful phase of your life, take charge of your vaginal health by arming yourself with these easy-to-use yet powerful techniques.

# Consulting Healthcare Professionals During Pregnancy

Although being pregnant is a wonderful and life-changing experience, there are certain difficulties and health issues that come with it. Your body goes through a number of physiological adjustments to help the foetus grow and thrive. These alterations frequently result in a higher chance of getting some illnesses, like yeast infections.

Pregnancy-related yeast infections are common because of altered hormone levels and increased vaginal discharge. If left untreated, yeast infections can become a cause for concern even though the majority of them are benign and easily cured. For this reason, seeking medical advice from medical specialists is essential when pregnant.

The first step in treating yeast infections during pregnancy is realising how crucial it is to consult a doctor. By speaking with medical specialists, you can obtain important medical information and advice. They are qualified to evaluate your particular circumstance and offer suitable therapy alternatives. This contributes to your baby's and your own wellbeing.

Knowing when to seek medical guidance is one of the most important parts of talking with healthcare professionals throughout pregnancy. Understanding the warning signs and symptoms of a yeast infection is crucial. These include burning, redness, swelling, itching, and irregular vaginal discharge. You should get medical help right away if you encounter any of these symptoms.

Seeking medical counsel becomes even more necessary in some instances, in addition to the symptoms listed above. In order to avoid complications, it is best to speak with medical specialists as soon as possible if you have previously experienced recurring yeast infections. Likewise, seeking medical advice from a physician is crucial if you have previously experienced immune system issues or have attempted over-the-counter remedies without results.

Pregnancy-related untreated yeast infections may have negative effects on the mother and the unborn child. If the infection is not treated, it may spread to other body parts and cause more serious issues. This may cause the mother to feel uncomfortable, have pain during sexual activity, and have trouble urinating. Additionally, it may result in postpartum issues and an elevated risk of infection during birth.

Furthermore, the growing foetus may be at risk from untreated yeast infections during pregnancy. Diaper rash or oral thrush may result from the infection sometimes being transferred to the newborn. Untreated yeast infections during pregnancy may also raise the chance of low birth weight and preterm delivery, according to some studies. These are grave problems that emphasise how crucial it is to consult a doctor in order to receive the right care.

I take a comprehensive and individualised approach to treating yeast infections during pregnancy as a healthcare provider. I firmly think that lifestyle changes, such as wearing breathable cotton underwear, practising good hygiene, and staying away from irritating feminine items, can make a significant impact. By taking these steps, you can help to prevent yeast infections and improve the general health of your vagina.

To help with the management of yeast infections, I also advise dietary adjustments in addition to lifestyle improvements. By adding probiotics to your diet, you can lower your chance of yeast overgrowth and help the vaginal flora return to its natural equilibrium. Foods high in probiotics include kefir, yoghurt, and fermented vegetables. Reducing the intake of processed foods and sugar is also crucial because these things can promote the growth of yeast.

Since stress can impair immunity and raise the risk of infections, controlling stress levels is especially essential during pregnancy. In order to help women deal with the psychological and emotional aspects of pregnancy, I frequently use counselling and psychology-related strategies in my practise. By offering assistance and imparting coping mechanisms, my goal is to enable women to take charge of their health and overall wellbeing.

In conclusion, seeking medical advice from professionals is crucial, particularly when it comes to treating yeast infections during pregnancy. For the sake of both the mother and the unborn child, it is critical to recognise the warning signs and symptoms of yeast infections, to know when to seek medical attention, and to be aware of the possible consequences of leaving an infection untreated. Through a comprehensive strategy that integrates dietary adjustments, lifestyle modifications, and counselling methods, we can guarantee that expectant mothers have the essential attention and assistance for comprehensive management of yeast infections. Recall that you should always put your health first and that consulting a doctor is the first step to a happy and healthy pregnancy.

# Chapter 10: Yeast Infections in Children and Infants

# Understanding Yeast Infections in Children and Infants

Let's first define yeast infections before getting into the specifics. The proliferation of a fungus called Candida is the cause of yeast infections, also referred to as candidiasis. Our bodies naturally contain this fungus, especially in regions like the mouth, skin, and gastrointestinal system. In most cases, having Candida does not have any negative effects. But some things can upset the delicate balance of microbes in the body, which can cause an overabundance of Candida and an infection.

Let's now concentrate on young children and babies. Although yeast infections can affect people of any age, they tend to affect younger people more frequently because of their immature immune systems. When the immune system is weak, as it frequently is in children and newborns, the risk of infection rises since the immune system is essential in controlling the population of Candida.

Common Sites of Infection:

Yeast infections in infants and toddlers can affect different parts of the body. Diaper rash is a frequent condition that arises from infections in the diaper area, which is one of the most prevalent sources of infection. This can be extremely irritating for the young children and is characterised by redness, swelling, and blisters in the diaper area. Diapers provide a great breeding habitat for Candida because of their warm, wet atmosphere.

Oral thrush is often the result of infection in the mouth. The tongue, inner cheeks, and roof of the mouth all have white, cottage cheese-like areas that are indicative of this illness. Oral thrush is more common in babies who use pacifiers or are bottle-fed because these products might host the Candida fungus.

Infections in children and newborns can also occur in the nails and scalp, as well as in skin folds like the armpits and neck. The youngster may experience discomfort as a result of redness, itching, and inflammation in these places.

Risk Factors:

Yeast infections in infants and toddlers can arise from a variety of causes. First off, as was already noted, they are more vulnerable to infections of all types, including yeast infections, due to their immature immune systems. Furthermore, the overgrowth of Candida can result from antibiotic use upsetting the body's normal microbial equilibrium. It is crucial to remember that, in order to reduce this danger, antibiotics should only be administered to children and newborns when absolutely necessary.

In addition, since the Candida fungus may readily grow on bottle-fed babies and pacifier-using newborns, these children are more susceptible to getting yeast infections, including oral thrush infection. Furthermore, the sugars in formula milk have the potential to promote Candida, raising the risk of infection even higher.

Complications:

Although yeast infections in infants and children are usually not thought to be dangerous, problems may arise if the illness is not treated. In severe situations, systemic fungal infections may result from the infection spreading to other parts of the body. Serious symptoms like fever, exhaustion, and organ damage may arise from this.

If left untreated, oral thrush can make it difficult for the infant to eat, which can result in inadequate nutrition and poor weight gain. Yeast infection-related diaper rash can be extremely unpleasant and uncomfortable for the infant, making changing diapers difficult for both the child and the parents.

In summary, a thorough understanding of yeast infections in kids and newborns is essential for efficient treatment and avoidance. We can take the required precautions to shield our children from the discomfort and possible harm caused by these fungal infections by identifying typical locations of infection, risk factors, and potential sequelae. We will look at a number of therapeutic and preventive approaches in the upcoming chapters that can be used to treat and prevent yeast infections in newborns and kids while also improving their general health and well-being.

# Preventive Measures and Hygiene Practices for Children

Candida infections, sometimes referred to as yeast infections, can affect the mouth, skin, and genitalia, among other parts of the body. Diaper rash is one of the most prevalent forms of yeast infections in children. It develops when the warm, wet atmosphere of a diaper provides the ideal conditions for yeast to grow.

Appropriate diapering practises, a consistent bathing schedule, and well-chosen clothing are crucial for preventing yeast infections in kids.

Diapering Techniques:

Using the right diapering practises is essential to keeping kids' yeast infections at bay. Here are a few crucial things to think about:

1. Frequently change diapers: It's crucial to change your child's diaper on a regular basis to keep the region dry and clean. Aim to change the diaper every few hours or as soon as it gets soiled because moisture might promote the growth of yeast.

2. Use breathable diapers: Choose breathable diapers, including those made of bamboo or cotton, as these promote greater air circulation and aid in keeping the diaper region dry. Steer clear of synthetic or overly tight diapers as they might retain moisture and foster the perfect habitat for the growth of yeast.

3. Avoid fragrance and harsh chemicals: Choose fragrance-free options for wipes and diapers. Strong chemicals and fragrances can irritate the sensitive skin around the diaper area, upsetting its natural equilibrium and increasing the risk of yeast infections.

4. Apply a protective barrier: Put a thin coating of petroleum jelly or diaper cream on your child's skin to act as a barrier between their skin and the diaper. By lowering friction and irritation, this may aid in stopping the growth of yeast.

Bathing Routines:

Another critical component in shielding kids from yeast infections is establishing a consistent bathing schedule. Here are some pointers to think about:

1. Use gentle, pH-balanced soaps: Select gentle, hypoallergenic soaps made especially for sensitive skin while giving your child a bath. Tough cleansers and soaps can upset the skin's normal pH balance, increasing the risk of yeast infections.

2. Pay special attention to the diaper area: Make sure your child's diaper region is completely cleaned and dried during bath time. After using a mild cleanser and warm water to gently wash the area, pat it dry with a soft cloth. Steer clear of rubbing or vigorous cleaning as this can aggravate the skin even more.

3. Avoid bubble baths: Although kids might like bubble baths, they can introduce possible allergens and upset the skin's natural equilibrium. Instead, to encourage relaxation without compromising the integrity of the skin, use plain water or a few drops of calming essential oils like chamomile or lavender.

4. Keep bath toys clean: Bacteria and yeast can be easily harboured by bath toys. After every usage, make sure to thoroughly wipe and dry them to avoid transferring dangerous bacteria onto your child's skin.

Clothing Choices:

Our children's wardrobe selections can also have a big impact on avoiding yeast infections. Here are some pointers to think about:

1. Choose breathable fabrics: Choose clothes made of breathable materials, such bamboo or cotton, as these promote greater airflow and keep the skin dry. Steer clear of synthetic or tight-fitting textiles as they might retain moisture and foster an environment that is favourable to the growth of yeast.

2. Avoid irritating materials: Certain textiles, like wool or some synthetic materials, have the potential to cause skin irritation and exacerbate yeast infections. Remain with materials that are soft, hypoallergenic, and kind to the skin.

3. Dress appropriately for the weather: Wear light-colored, loose-fitting clothing in warmer weather to improve ventilation and reduce moisture accumulation. Wear layers of clothes in cooler weather to avoid being too hot or perspiring too much.

4. Wash clothing with care: Use gentle, fragrance-free detergents free of harsh chemicals to wash your child's clothes. Dryer sheets and fabric softeners should not be used because they might irritate skin and upset the body's natural equilibrium.

Parents and other caregivers can drastically lower their child's chance of developing yeast infections by putting these preventive measures and hygiene habits into practise. But keep in mind that each child is different, so what works for one might not work for another. If you are unsure about your child's hygiene regimen or have any concerns, speak with your paediatrician or other healthcare practitioner.

Teaching kids proper hygienic habits at a young age is crucial, in addition to these preventive steps. Urge children to routinely wash their hands, particularly before meals and after using the restroom. Instruct them on appropriate wiping methods, with a focus on front-to-back wiping, to stop bacteria from moving from the anus to the vaginal or urine entrance.

Additionally, it's critical to teach kids the value of boundaries and personal space. Promote open discussion about any pain or discomfort in the genital area and emphasise the need of getting medical attention from a qualified healthcare provider or trusted adult.

Overall, we can lay a solid foundation for our kids' long-term health and wellbeing by implementing these preventative measures and hygiene practises into their everyday routines. We enable them to take charge of their own health and lower the risk of yeast infections and other common illnesses by arming them with the information and resources they need to maintain proper hygiene practises.

# Safe Treatment Options for Children and Infants

Since children's bodies are still developing and their immune systems are not as strong as adults', treating yeast infections in these patients might be difficult. However, these infections can be efficiently managed and the little ones who are suffering can be given relief with the appropriate strategy and thoughtful thinking.

Using topical creams is one of the most popular ways to treat yeast infections in kids and babies. These topical lotions relieve symptoms and eradicate yeast when applied directly to the afflicted region. Because their skin is more delicate and prone to irritation, babies and children should always use creams that are especially made for them. Antifungal creams containing miconazole or clotrimazole are among the over-the-counter alternatives; these medications are usually safe for use in youngsters. Before administering any medication to a child, it is best to speak with a healthcare provider, since they may offer advice based on the child's particular needs and medical background.

Oral drugs may be required in certain instances to treat infants' and children's yeast infections, especially if the illness is more severe or has spread to other body regions. A licenced healthcare provider can prescribe oral antifungal drugs, like fluconazole, to help treat the yeast infection internally. The usage of these drugs should only be done so under the direction and supervision of a healthcare provider due to the possibility of negative effects.

There are a number of potentially safe and efficient natural treatments for yeast infections in kids and babies. Probiotics, for instance, can help prevent the accumulation of yeast in the body and restore the natural balance of microorganisms in it. Probiotics can be taken as supplements or through specific foods like kefir or yoghurt. Before beginning any new supplement regimen, it is imperative to select a probiotic that is especially made for babies and children and to speak with a medical practitioner.

Coconut oil is another all-natural treatment that works well for treating infants' and children's yeast infections. The antifungal qualities of coconut oil can aid in eliminating the yeast and alleviating the symptoms. For a calming and restorative effect, it can be added to bath water or administered directly to the affected area. To make sure there are no negative responses, it is crucial to conduct a patch test on a small section of skin before using a natural medicine extensively.

It is critical to address the underlying causes of yeast infections in children and infants in addition to these treatment choices. These may include using antibiotics excessively, wearing clothes that is too tight, or practising improper hygiene. You may aid in preventing further infections by ensuring that the kid wears loose-fitting, breathable clothing and by putting appropriate hygiene measures into practise, such as frequent bathing and gentle cleansing of the afflicted areas.

It's also crucial to remember that candida infections in kids and newborns can occasionally indicate underlying medical conditions like diabetes or compromised immune systems. It's critical to speak with a healthcare provider for additional assessment and direction if your child keeps getting yeast infections or if the symptoms don't get better after therapy.

In summary, a cautious and customised strategy is needed to treat yeast infections in kids and newborns. We can put into practise safe and efficient treatment solutions by taking into account their distinct physiology and potential dangers. To determine the best course of action for your child's unique needs, whether it be topical creams, oral drugs, or natural therapies, it is crucial to speak with a healthcare provider. We can help our children overcome these infections and improve their general health and well-being with the right care and preventive measures.

# When to Consult a Pediatric Healthcare Professional

I firmly believe in promoting holistic healthcare and wellness as a medical doctor and health and wellness coach. It's critical to recognise when to seek the advice of a paediatric healthcare provider when it comes to treating yeast infections in kids and babies. I will walk you through the symptoms and indicators in this chapter that call for a consultation so that your children can receive quick and effective medical care.

Yeast infections can cause a variety of symptoms in different parts of the body in children and infants. Diaper rash, oral thrush, and vaginal yeast infections are a few of the most typical forms of yeast infections in kids. A healthcare provider may be needed in some circumstances, even if some cases can be treated with over-the-counter medications and home cures.

The severity and persistence of symptoms is one of the first indicators that you may need to see a doctor. For example, you should see a paediatric healthcare provider if your child's yeast infection does not go better after a week of taking over-the-counter remedies, or if the symptoms get worse even while your child is maintaining good hygiene. In order to address the underlying source of the illness, they can perform a more thorough assessment of the problem and may suggest prescription drugs or other forms of treatment.

The child's age is a crucial consideration as well. Infants have sensitive immune systems that are still developing, especially those under three months old. Therefore, in this age range, any indications or symptoms of a yeast infection should be taken seriously and should prompt a visit with a medical practitioner. It's also important to get medical attention right away since babies who are prematurely delivered or who have other underlying medical issues may be more vulnerable to serious yeast infections.

When it comes to infant and toddler yeast infections, there are some telltale indications and symptoms that should never be disregarded. It is crucial that you get in touch with a paediatric healthcare provider right away if you observe any of the following:

1. Persistent or recurrent diaper rash: While diaper rash is typical in babies, it may be a sign of a yeast infection if it doesn't go away in spite of good cleanliness and frequent diaper changes. A medical expert can provide an accurate diagnosis and suggest the best course of action to ease your child's discomfort.

2. White patches in the mouth: A fungal illness called oral thrush can cause white patches on an infant's tongue, cheeks, or roof of the mouth. In order to guarantee proper treatment and stop the illness from spreading, it's critical that you speak with a healthcare provider as soon as you discover these patches.

3. Vaginal itching, redness, and discharge: Vaginal yeast infections are less prevalent in youngsters, although they can still happen, especially in older girls who have entered puberty. It's critical to seek medical assistance if your child complains of vaginal itching, redness, or unusual discharge in order to rule out any underlying causes and administer the appropriate treatment.

4. Unexplained fever or systemic symptoms: Occasionally, systemic symptoms like fever, irritability, or tiredness can be caused by yeast infections. These signs could point to a more serious infection that needs to be treated right now. It's critical to take these symptoms seriously and to see a doctor right away.

5. Difficulty feeding or swallowing: It is imperative that you seek medical attention if your infant exhibits fussiness or refuses to eat along with difficulties with feeding or swallowing. These signs could point to an oral thrush infection, which can cause your infant to have painful or uncomfortable feeding experiences.

The management of yeast infections in infants and children depends heavily on prompt and proper medical intervention. You can make sure that your children receive the care and attention that they require by speaking with a paediatric healthcare expert. Healthcare providers may recommend preventive measures, such as keeping good hygiene, eating a healthy diet, and changing one's lifestyle, in addition to prescribing medicine to treat yeast infections.

As a caretaker, never forget how important it is to believe your gut. Do not hesitate to seek medical advice from a specialist if something seems strange or if your child's symptoms do not seem to improve with at-home treatments. Seeking prompt medical attention can help avoid any potential consequences or long-term repercussions in addition to addressing the current infection. A paediatric healthcare professional can help you manage your child's yeast infection and is the person to call when your child's health and well-being are at risk.

We'll look at some practical lifestyle changes and at-home remedies in the upcoming chapter that can support prescription medications and help shield kids and babies from yeast infections. When combined, these tactics will enable you to become an expert in treating yeast infections and safeguard your children's general health. Watch this space for insightful analysis and useful tips to accelerate your journey to conquering yeast infections.

# Chapter 11: Emotional Support and Mental Well-being

# Addressing the Emotional Impact of Yeast Infections

It might be startling and upsetting for someone to learn they have a yeast infection for the first time. Itching, burning, and discharge are a few of the irritating and life-interrupting symptoms. The person experiencing this physical discomfort may feel unclean, disgusting, and self-conscious about their body, which can swiftly escalate into mental distress.

Frustration is a typical feeling that people with yeast infections experience. It can be very irritating to deal with the ongoing pain and annoyance, especially when it seems like there isn't a quick fix. This aggravation frequently results in hopelessness and despair as the person questions whether they will ever be able to find relief.

Another prevalent feeling among people with yeast infections is embarrassment. Discussing or addressing symptoms like vaginal discharge and itching in public might be awkward. A person's illness may cause them to feel stigmatised or ashamed, which can lower their self-esteem and confidence. It is critical to keep in mind that yeast infections are a common and treatable illness, and that asking for assistance or being honest about your symptoms doesn't indicate shame or embarrassment.

Aside from irritation and shame, people with yeast infections can often feel anxious and doubtful of themselves. They can doubt their own personal hygiene habits or be concerned about their reputation. These unfavourable feelings and ideas can have a serious detrimental effect on one's mental health and make it more challenging to manage the infection's physical symptoms.

In order to effectively address the psychological effects of yeast infections, a holistic strategy emphasising mental and physical health is needed. The following techniques can assist people in controlling and reducing the psychological toll that yeast infections have on them:

1. Education and awareness: Some of the guilt and embarrassment related to yeast infections can be reduced by realising that they are a common and treatable ailment. Learn about the signs, symptoms, and available treatments for yeast infections, and then impart this knowledge to family members or close friends who could be going through a similar experience.

2. Self-care and relaxation techniques: Managing your health both mentally and physically is crucial when treating a yeast infection. Take care of yourself by doing things like taking warm baths, taking meditation classes, deep breathing exercises, or relaxing pastimes. Engaging in these hobbies can lower stress and improve general wellbeing.

3. Seek support: Seeking assistance from those who comprehend and have gone through comparable struggles can be beneficial. Making an online or in-person connection with a support group can offer a secure setting for you to express your feelings, exchange experiences, and get advice from those going through comparable circumstances. Having a therapist, family member, or friend's support can also help manage the emotional effects of yeast infections.

4. Practice self-compassion: It is imperative that you treat yourself with kindness and compassion during this period. Emotional anguish can be aggravated further by self-blame and negative self-talk. Practice saying self-compassionate things such, "I am not alone in this," "I am taking care of myself as best I can," and "I deserve love and support."

5. Communicate openly with your healthcare provider: It is imperative to talk to your healthcare professional if you discover that the psychological effects of your yeast infection are having a substantial negative impact on your mental health. If necessary, they can provide you with direction, encouragement, and possibly even a referral to a mental health specialist.

Recall that feelings are a legitimate and necessary component of the recovery process. It's critical to allow oneself to feel and express these feelings without guilt. People can improve their general well-being and get relief from the emotional and physical effects of yeast infections by treating and managing the emotional impact of the condition.

# Seeking Emotional Support From Loved Ones

It is normal to feel a range of emotions when dealing with a yeast infection or any other health issue, from annoyance and rage to melancholy and hopelessness. Coping with the physical and emotional components of the disease can be difficult due to these intense feelings. It is essential to navigate these feelings and find the strength to effectively manage the infection by asking loved ones for emotional assistance.

Acknowledging and understanding that you need emotional support is one of the first steps toward getting it. Asking for assistance can be challenging for many people, particularly those who are used to being independent. But it's crucial to realise that asking for help is an empowering act of self-care rather than a show of weakness. Recognizing that you require emotional support indicates that you are taking an active role in your general wellbeing.

It's important to communicate well when asking loved ones for emotional support. It's critical that you communicate your requirements, wants, and feelings in an understandable and direct way. Communicate honestly and openly, expressing your feelings and experiences without worrying about being judged. Indicate exactly what kind of help you require, if it's just someone to listen, give you advise, or just be there to console you.

Creating a network of support is another crucial step in getting emotional support. In addition to the priceless support that friends, family, and loved ones may offer, it's critical to think about the options of joining support groups or getting professional assistance. Support groups offer a special setting where people can interact with others who are going through comparable difficulties. These clubs can provide a very consoling sense of understanding, camaraderie, and shared experiences.

Apart from joining support groups, getting expert assistance can also be helpful. Like myself, a health and wellness coach may offer direction and encouragement along with useful tactics for handling the psychological effects of a yeast infection. They possess the know-how and experience to assist you in putting self-help, coping mechanisms, and lifestyle changes into practise that will improve your mental health.

It's critical to keep in mind that providing emotional support requires reciprocation. It is crucial to ask loved ones for help, but it is just as crucial to be a source of support for them. Relationships involving emotional support should be mutually beneficial and reciprocal. You can build a network of people who care about your general well-being and are available to offer you the emotional support you require anytime you need it by fostering and preserving these relationships.

It's crucial to understand, though, that not every loved one will be able to provide you the emotional support you need. Some others might not fully comprehend your illness, or they might be experiencing emotional difficulties of their own. It's critical to understand these constraints and, if need, look for assistance elsewhere. This could include contacting close friends, taking up enjoyable hobbies or pastimes, or even thinking about going to therapy or counselling.

Furthermore, it's critical to keep in mind that receiving emotional support is a continuous process. It is a continual process that needs constant attention and support. Communicate your wants and sentiments to your loved ones on a regular basis. Together, celebrate the victories and advancements, but also be honest about the obstacles and setbacks.

In summary, it is imperative to seek emotional support from friends, family, and loved ones in order to manage the emotional burden of a yeast infection, or any other medical issue. It is a powerful self-care practise that has a big impact on your general wellbeing. Develop a support system, communicate effectively, and show that you're willing to get expert assistance when you need it. Keep in mind that emotional support is mutual, so asking for and providing support for your loved ones is just as vital as giving them to you. Lastly, keep in mind that providing emotional support is a continual process that calls for nurturing and constant effort. You may effectively control your yeast infection and achieve emotional equilibrium by accepting this journey and getting help when required.

# Coping With Anxiety and Stress

Practical Techniques for Coping with Anxiety and Stress Related to Yeast Infections

As a physician and health and wellness coach, I have worked with many patients who not only battle with the outward manifestations of yeast infections but also deal with a great deal of stress and anxiety because of their illness. These infections can cause excruciating pain, discomfort, and itching, which can be extremely difficult to deal with emotionally and psychologically. I'll give you useful coping mechanisms and resources in this chapter to help you manage the tension and worry that frequently accompany yeast infections.

1. Relaxation exercises:

Relaxation techniques are a great method to ease tension and encourage serenity. You can control the mental, physical, and even yeast infection-related symptoms of stress with the use of these approaches. Deep breathing is a useful technique for relaxing. Close your eyes, choose a comfortable place to sit or lie down, and inhale deeply and slowly. Feel the tension in your body release as you take deep breaths with your nose and feel your abdomen rise. Then, slowly release the breath through your mouth. Continue doing this for a few minutes, or until you start to feel more at ease.

Progressive muscle relaxation is an additional helpful relaxation method. Tense the muscles in your toes first, and then gradually move up your body, tensing and relaxing each muscle group as you go. You may encourage a state of both physical and mental relaxation by paying attention to your body's sensations and intentionally releasing tension.

2. Mindfulness practices:

The practise of mindfulness involves focusing attention on the current moment without passing judgement. It's simple to let negative ideas and feelings to take over while you're experiencing the physical discomfort associated with yeast infections. You can lessen your stress and anxiety by using mindfulness to help you turn your attention from your symptoms to the here and now.

You can experiment with body scan meditation as one mindfulness technique. Taking a comfortable posture on the floor, focus on each part of your body, working your way up to your head from your toes. Without passing judgement, take note of any tensions or uncomfortable spots and give yourself permission to just be in the moment. Developing a non-reactive and accepting mindset will help you lessen the emotional pain that comes with yeast infections.

3. Stress reduction strategies:

Although stress is an inevitable part of life, it is important to manage it efficiently in order to maintain general wellbeing, particularly when coping with the difficulties associated with a yeast infection. The anxiety and tension related to this illness can be considerably reduced by implementing stress reduction techniques.

Exercise is a useful tactic for reducing stress. Frequent physical activity helps lower stress chemicals like cortisol in addition to encouraging the release of endorphins. Make it a point to fit in enjoyable hobbies like yoga, swimming, or walking as part of your everyday schedule.

Exercise is not the only important factor in stress reduction; self-care activities are also essential. Spend some time relaxing and having fun with the things you enjoy doing for yourself. This can be using aromatherapy, having a warm bath, enjoying some relaxing music, or going outside. Making self-care a priority can help you live a more balanced and tranquil life and lessen the negative effects of stress on your mental and emotional health.

4. Seek support:

It's crucial to keep in mind that you're not alone when dealing with a yeast infection, even though it might be a lonely and isolated experience. Seek out the assistance of dependable family members, friends, or medical experts who can offer support and understanding. It can be incredibly relieving to discuss your thoughts and concerns with someone who understands your circumstances and can support you in overcoming the emotional difficulties brought on by yeast infections.

Joining online forums or support groups devoted to managing yeast infections can also be a great help. These platforms provide a secure environment where users can interact with others going through comparable situations, exchange advice, and pick up coping mechanisms. Creating a network of support can give you a feeling of empowerment and belonging, which will further lower your stress and anxiety levels.

Conclusion:

Although treating yeast infections' physical symptoms is crucial, it's also critical to address the emotional and psychological toll that this illness can have. You can effectively manage the anxiety and tension associated with yeast infections by implementing mindfulness exercises, relaxation techniques, and stress reduction tactics into your daily routine. To promote resilience and a sense of well-being, never forget to ask for help when you need it and to practise self-care. You can take a more comprehensive approach to managing yeast infections by taking back control of your mental and emotional well-being with the help of these useful strategies and resources.

# Mental Well-being and Self-Care Practices

We must first examine the idea of self-care in order to fully comprehend the relationship between mental health and yeast infections. Taking care of our bodily well-being is only one aspect of self-care. It entails taking care of our mental, emotional, and spiritual needs. It involves striking a balance in our life and setting aside time to attend to our own needs.

Self-care rituals are private routines that enhance wellbeing and assist in reestablishing equilibrium in our life. Depending on the needs and tastes of the individual, they might take on many forms. It could be a yoga or meditation routine in the morning for some people. For some, it can be writing in a journal, having a soothing bath, or just going outside. The secret is to engage in things that make us happy and revitalised.

In addition, positive affirmations are very important for fostering mental and emotional health. We tell ourselves these empowering affirmations to dispel unfavourable ideas and perceptions. Affirmations are an effective technique for good mental development and mind reprogramming. They can support a sense of wellbeing, lessen tension, and help with self-confidence building. Positive affirmations for mental health include things like "I am tough and capable of overcoming any hardship that comes my way" and "I am worthy of love and happiness."

Managing yeast infections also requires engaging in activities that support mental and emotional wellness. Anxiety, despair, and stress can impair immunity, leaving the body more vulnerable to diseases. Finding constructive outlets to reduce stress and improve mental health is so essential.

Studies have indicated that engaging in practises like physical activity, practising mindful meditation, and deep breathing might lower stress levels and enhance mental health. Frequent exercise releases endorphins, the feel-good hormones that can help reduce the symptoms of depression and anxiety, in addition to improving physical health. Mind-calming and stress-reduction practises that involve deep breathing, such diaphragmatic breathing, can be beneficial. Contrarily, mindfulness meditation entails concentrating on and embracing the current moment without passing judgement. It has been demonstrated that this technique lessens the signs of stress, anxiety, and sadness.

It's crucial to develop self-compassion and self-acceptance techniques in addition to self-care routines and encouraging statements. People who have yeast infections frequently experience feelings of shame or embarrassment, which can result in self-criticism and negative self-talk. It's critical to keep in mind that yeast infections are widespread and do not determine our value as people. For our mental and emotional health, we must learn to accept our bodies, the difficulties we confront, and to be kind to ourselves.

In order to manage mental health, coping mechanisms are also essential. It is crucial to establish coping mechanisms in order to manage the mental and physical discomfort brought on by yeast infections. This can involve asking for help from close friends and family or joining a support group, taking part in enjoyable and distracting activities, and practising relaxation methods like progressive muscle relaxation or guided imagery.

In summary, self-care routines and mental health are important components of controlling yeast infections. Readers can learn self-care practises, positive affirmations, and activities that support mental and emotional wellness by examining the relationship between these two characteristics. People can improve the way they manage their yeast infections and build resilience and general well-being by adopting these strategies into their daily life. In my capacity as a physician and health and wellness coach, I strongly advise everyone to put their mental and emotional well-being first and to fully utilise self-care as they work toward managing their yeast infections.

# Chapter 12: Integrating Yeast Infection Management Into Daily Life

# Time Management and Prioritization

Introduction:

Taking care of a yeast infection might be difficult since it calls both self-care and medication. Finding the time to put our health first can often feel daunting in today's hectic society. But people can make a balanced plan that lets them take care of their yeast infection and other obligations at the same time by using efficient time management strategies.

The Importance of Time Management:

For those who are controlling yeast infections, time management skills are essential. When balancing obligations to their family, job, and other commitments, it helps avoid ignoring their health demands. A systematic approach to time management can help people make sure they have adequate time for treatment and self-care, which lowers the risk of chronic or recurrent yeast infections.

1. Assessing Priorities:

Prioritizing is the first stage in time management. It entails determining which responsibilities and tasks are necessary and which ones can be transferred or dropped. Treating and taking care of oneself must come first when controlling a yeast infection. People who understand the importance of their health are better able to set aside the time needed to care for themselves.

2. Creating a Schedule:

After priorities have been determined, it's critical to develop a plan that fits all obligations, including treatment and self-care. There should be designated times on this plan for things like taking medications, taking care of oneself, and scheduling doctor's visits. Through the integration of these activities into a regimented schedule, patients can guarantee adherence to their treatment regimen.

3. Time Blocking:

Allocating distinct time blocks for various activities throughout the day is known as time blocking. Time blocking can be a useful tool for people with yeast infections to make sure they set aside specific time for treatment and self-care. People are able to establish a daily schedule that accommodates their health requirements without interfering with other commitments by setting aside particular times.

4. Eliminating Time Wasters:

In order to optimise their time, people need to recognise and get rid of activities that take up unnecessary time. This could entail cutting back on time spent on social media, pointless gatherings, and other ineffective activities. People can efficiently control their yeast infection by freeing up more time for self-care and treatment by getting rid of time wasters.

5. Delegation and Support:

Taking care of a yeast infection shouldn't be done alone. To lessen the load, it's critical to ask for help from close ones and assign certain tasks to others. This could include asking a spouse to help with housework, asking a friend or family member to pick up groceries, or assigning coworkers to do work-related activities. By dividing the workload, people can free up more time for therapy and self-care, which will ultimately enhance their general wellbeing.

6. Effective Communication:

When prioritising health and managing time, effective communication is essential. It's critical to be transparent about the need to set aside time for treatment and self-care with family, coworkers, and employers. People can ensure they have the time needed to effectively manage their yeast infection by fostering understanding and support by setting clear expectations and boundaries.

7. Flexibility and Adaptability:

Even though we make an effort to maintain a well-organized routine, life frequently presents us with unforeseen difficulties. Maintaining flexibility and adaptability is crucial when it comes to time management and health prioritisation. It is simpler to deal with unforeseen events without sacrificing self-care and therapy when one is ready to modify schedules as needed.

Conclusion:

Those who are controlling yeast infections must have strong time management and prioritisation skills. People can design a balanced schedule that prioritises self-care and treatment while still fulfilling their other responsibilities by putting the strategies covered in this subchapter into practise. You should always prioritise your health and well-being, and you can make sure you give yourself the time and care you need to treat and avoid yeast infections by practising efficient time management.

# Incorporating Healthy Habits Into Daily Routine

"You are what you repeatedly do. Excellence, then, is not an act but a habit." - Aristotle

Maintaining a healthy lifestyle involves more than just sticking to a short-term, rigid diet or exercise schedule. It involves consistently making decisions that promote your general well-being. I'll walk you through incorporating healthy behaviours into your everyday routine in this chapter. I'll give you all the tools and tactics you need to make long-lasting changes, from workout and diet planning to self-care and relaxing methods.

Exercise

To keep your health at its best, you must engage in regular physical activity. It lowers your chance of getting heart disease and diabetes, among other chronic illnesses, in addition to aiding with weight management. Regular exercise has also been demonstrated to boost energy, improve mental health, and improve general wellbeing.

1.1 Finding an Exercise Routine That Works for You

Finding an activity you enjoy doing is the first step towards implementing fitness into your regular routine. Whether it's yoga, dancing, swimming, or jogging, pick an activity that makes you happy and eager to move your body. Try out a variety of workouts until you discover which ones work best for you.

1.2 Scheduling Your Workouts

After determining your favourite type of exercise, it's critical to establish a regular routine. Set aside specified periods for your workouts every day or every week, and treat them as appointments that cannot be cancelled. This will assist you in putting your health first and ensuring that working out is an essential part of your everyday schedule.

1.3 Breaking up Sedentary Time

It's critical to break up extended periods of sitting or inactivity throughout the day in addition to engaging in regular exercise. To remind yourself to get up and walk every hour, think about setting a timer. This could be practising some basic exercises, going for a little walk, or stretching. Your productivity and cognitive performance will both increase and your physical health will be enhanced by these brief vacations.

Meal Planning

Healthy eating is the cornerstone of good health. You can guarantee that you have access to wholesome food selections that promote your general well-being and nourish your body by organising your meals in advance.

2.1 Create a Weekly Meal Plan

Make a weekly meal plan that consists of a range of foods that are high in nutrients. This can help you avoid making rash dietary decisions that could not support your health objectives, in addition to saving you time and money. Make entire foods like fruits, vegetables, lean proteins, whole grains, and healthy fats the focal point of your meals.

2.2 Batch Cooking and Meal Prepping

Think about meal planning and batch cooking to make healthy eating more accessible. Set up a few hours once a week to prepare and cook greater amounts of food that can be quickly refrigerated or saved for later use. This will guarantee that you always have wholesome meals on hand while saving you time and effort.

2.3 Mindful Eating

Healthy eating practises involve more than just what you eat; they also entail how you eat. Take a conscious approach to eating by focusing on the tastes, textures, and feelings of your meal. Eat mindfully, relishing every taste, and giving yourself the opportunity to enjoy eating to the fullest. This will assist you in improving digestion and reducing overeating in addition to assisting you in making more thoughtful food choices.

Relaxation Techniques

Finding times of calm and relaxation in today's hectic environment is crucial for general wellbeing. Including relaxation techniques in your daily routine can aid with stress management, enhance the quality of your sleep, and foster inner calm.

3.1 Breathing Exercises

Exercises including deep breathing are an easy yet powerful technique to put yourself in a relaxed condition right away. Close your eyes, choose a comfortable spot to sit or lie down, and inhale deeply through your nose. As you breathe in into your lungs, feel your tummy rise. Breathe out slowly through your mouth to let go of any stress or anxiety. For several minutes, repeat this exercise while concentrating on your breathing pattern and putting your rushing thoughts aside.

3.2 Meditation

One of the most effective ways to calm your mind and develop a strong sense of inner peace is through meditation. Locate a peaceful area where you may sit comfortably without being bothered. Shut your eyes and focus on your breathing or any preferred mantra. Without passing judgement, let your thoughts come and go. When they do, gently return your attention back to the here and now. As you grow more accustomed to the practise, progressively extend the amount of time you spend meditating each day from a few minutes at first.

3.3 Incorporating Self-Care Practices

Maintaining your general well-being requires that you make self-care routines a daily part of your routine. Find things to do that make you happy and feel nourished, whether it's taking a warm bath, journaling, engaging in a hobby, or going outside. Prioritize your own well-being and set aside time each week for rest and indulgence.

In conclusion, it may not always be simple to incorporate healthy behaviours into your daily schedule, but the effort is well worth it.

You may change your life and reach your best health and well-being by making deliberate decisions and continuously engaging in healthy behaviours. Recall that progress, not perfection, is what matters. Commence modest, remain steady, and acknowledge each small victory on the path to a better, happier you.

# Managing Work and Social Life With Yeast Infections

It can be difficult to manage yeast infections both physically and psychologically. It has the potential to interfere with work and social interactions, among other elements of daily life. As a physician and health and wellness coach, I know how crucial it is to strike a balance between taking care of your infections and carrying on with a happy life. I'll be sharing tips in this subchapter to assist you deal with yeast infections and still prioritise your health while managing your social and professional lives.

When it comes to managing your professional and social life while suffering from yeast infections, effective communication is essential. It's critical to discuss your issue honestly and freely with friends, coworkers, and superiors. Being open and honest about your circumstances might help you feel less stressed and make it easier for others to support you. People are often sympathetic and understanding.

It's important to talk about your situation with your immediate supervisor or the human resources department when it comes to your work life. They can provide remote work choices, flexible scheduling, or even shorter work hours to help meet your demands. It's crucial for your health to take breaks to deal with symptoms or go to doctor's visits, and having an honest discussion about your requirements can help make this happen.

It's crucial to let your coworkers know what you require. For instance, it could be beneficial to request a chair that is more ergonomically comfortable if your yeast infection is causing you pain or discomfort. This can reduce physical stress on your body and increase productivity at work.

Setting limits is crucial for managing your job and social life when you have yeast infections, in addition to effective communication.

Stress levels can be lowered and symptom exacerbations can be avoided by developing the ability to say no and giving self-care first priority. It's critical to understand your limitations and avoid going overboard.

Delegating work, cutting back on burden, or even taking the odd day off when needed are all examples of setting boundaries in the workplace. Establishing an atmosphere that promotes your general well-being can be achieved by being transparent about your constraints with your manager and coworkers.

It's critical to emphasise self-care and pay attention to your body in social situations. Refusing an invitation to an event or gathering that could exacerbate your symptoms or create discomfort is totally appropriate. Informing your loved ones and friends about your illness can make it easier for them to see why you need to put self-care first.

It can also be helpful to find different ways to socialise. Think about planning more private events or spending time in a more relaxing and quiet setting with your loved ones. By doing this, you can continue to take care of your health and your social life.

Another important part of managing your professional and social life while dealing with yeast infections is asking for help when you need it. It is crucial to keep in mind that you are not alone on this trip. Getting help from friends, family, or even support groups can be very beneficial in overcoming the difficulties and feelings associated with having a chronic illness such as yeast infections.

Inform your loved ones about your illness by reaching out to them. Talk about your wants, worries, and experiences. Having someone listen to you while you talk can sometimes be a huge relief. Having individuals who understand and support you can have a big impact on how you manage your social and professional lives.

Joining online forums or support groups catering to people with yeast infections could also be a source of comfort. These areas offer a forum for exchanging advice, coping mechanisms, and experiences.

Making connections with people who are experiencing similar things to you can be quite empowering and reduce feelings of loneliness.

Think about consulting with a therapist or counsellor who specialises in chronic conditions in addition to getting help from your loved ones and participating in support groups. They can offer you coping mechanisms, support you through any emotional difficulties, and provide insightful advice on how to successfully balance your social and professional lives.

In summary, good communication, establishing limits, and asking for help when needed are all necessary for balancing work and social life while dealing with yeast infections. Having frank conversations about your illness with coworkers, managers, and friends can help foster a supportive atmosphere that meets your requirements. Maintaining your general well-being requires prioritising self-care and setting boundaries in social and professional contexts. Throughout your journey, getting help from loved ones, support groups, and mental health specialists can be quite beneficial. Remind yourself that you are not alone in this and that you can successfully manage your social and professional lives while dealing with yeast infections provided you have the correct tools and assistance.

# Embracing Self-Compassion and Acceptance

Society has overemphasised conforming to a certain ideal and reaching perfection for far too long. Images of ideal bodies that have been photoshopped and polished to perfection are all around us. It is taught to us that any departure from this norm is a defect that has to be covered up and fixed immediately. This unachievable norm has permeated the healthcare industry, fostering a climate of guilt and self-blame when dealing with medical conditions like yeast infections.

However, I'm here to inform you that this way of thinking won't help you manage yeast infections. Accepting and practising self-compassion and acceptance is the first step toward real healing and wellbeing. It's about realising that you are worthy of love, compassion, and understanding and that your situation does not define you.

In order to manage yeast infections, readers will learn the value of self-compassion and acceptance. They will also learn how to accept their particular situation and take care of themselves without feeling guilty or judged. It is about realising that you are not alone on this trip and that a great number of others have gone through comparable struggles and found comfort in accepting their own path.

Studies have indicated that those who engage in self-compassion practises report feeling better mentally and emotionally. They are more adept at overcoming obstacles, navigating life's ups and downs, and developing a general sense of fulfilment and happiness. Self-compassion can make all the difference when it comes to treating yeast infections.

Imagine if you could treat your yeast infection with the same consideration and tenderness that you would show to a loved one going through a trying period. Instead of seeing your body as an enemy that betrays you at every flare-up, picture it as a vessel that needs gentle attention and nutrition. This mental change can have a profound effect on controlling yeast infections as well as developing a better connection with your body and yourself.

But with an illness that can feel so crippling and infuriating, how can you start to embrace self-compassion and acceptance? Recognizing that your path is distinct and legitimate and that your feelings and experiences are deserving of acknowledgement and comprehension is the first step. It involves granting oneself permission to put self-care first, to look for help and direction, and to let go of any guilt or judgement that may have been plaguing you for an excessive amount of time.

The practise of mindfulness is a potent technique for developing acceptance and self-compassion. Being mindful is focusing your attention on the here and now, judgment-free. Instead of becoming sucked into your thoughts and feelings, it enables you to watch them with love and curiosity. You are able to develop compassion and self-awareness through practising mindfulness.

Being aware of your body's demands and cues can help you manage yeast infections by helping you tune in to it. It can support you in making decisions regarding your lifestyle and health as well as assist you see the early warning indicators of an approaching flare-up. It can also give you a place to go through and manage any emotions that surface while you deal with the difficulties of treating yeast infections.

Letting go of comparisons and irrational expectations is an essential part of accepting self-compassion and acceptance. Comparing oneself to others is a common mistake, particularly in the social media age when it looks like everyone has everything together. However, each person's path is different, so what works for one person could not work for another.

This includes understanding that your treatment approach may be different from others when it comes to managing yeast infections. It entails accepting that obstacles are a normal part of the healing process and that it requires time and patience. It entails allowing yourself to look for supplementary and alternative methods that speak to you instead of mindlessly adhering to the newest craze or fashion.

Recall that addressing physical symptoms alone is not enough to manage yeast infections; you also need to take care of your body, mind, and spirit. It involves combining coping mechanisms, self-help tactics, counselling and psychology-related procedures, food and diet planning, lifestyle adjustments, and alternative and complementary forms of self-care. It's about putting your entire health first and figuring out what suits you the best.

To sum up, accepting oneself and practising self-compassion and acceptance is crucial to controlling yeast infections. It's about realising that no matter how healthy you are, you are valuable and worthy. It involves developing self-compassion and empathy as well as a sense of calm and fortitude in the face of adversity. Thus, inhale deeply and release the guilt and self-judgment. Your compass for a happier, healthier, and more fulfilled life is accepting self-compassion and acceptance. You are on a journey towards total yeast infection control.

# Chapter 13: Yeast Infections and Mental Health

# Yeast Infections and Mood Disorders

In my capacity as a physician and health and wellness coach, I have assisted many patients who have been dealing with mood problems and yeast infections. I have looked into the studies to learn more about the relationship between the two as I have observed it over the years. I hope to clarify the effects of yeast overgrowth on mental health in this subchapter and offer symptom management techniques.

Let's start by examining the effects of yeast overgrowth on the body in order to better comprehend the connection between yeast infections and mood problems. Candida albicans is a type of yeast that can cause candidiasis when it overproliferates in the body. Numerous variables, including a weakened immune system, a diet high in sugar and refined carbohydrates, hormonal changes, or long-term use of antibiotics, might contribute to this overgrowth.

The gut is where yeast overgrowth has one of the biggest effects. Because of its intimate relationship to mental health, the gut is frequently referred to as the "second brain." Trillions of bacteria reside there, some of which are helpful for digestion and nutrient absorption. Nevertheless, the delicate balance of these bacteria is upset when Candida overpopulates the gut, resulting in an imbalance known as dysbiosis.

Leaky gut syndrome is a condition where toxins are released into the circulation as a result of dysbiosis brought on by yeast overgrowth. This illness causes the intestinal lining to become permeable to foreign substances and undigested food particles, which then enters the circulation and causes an inflammatory reaction. The body, especially the brain, may be greatly impacted by this persistent inflammation.

Numerous research have demonstrated a clear correlation between mental health conditions like depression, anxiety, and bipolar disorder and gut dysbiosis. The so-called "gut-brain axis" is essential for controlling behaviour and mood. The production and availability of

164

neurotrasmitters involved in mood regulation, such as serotonin, dopamine, and GABA, can be impacted when the balance of gut bacteria is upset.

Furthermore, there may be a direct impact on brain function from the toxins generated by Candida overgrowth. Certain toxins, like acetaldehyde, prevent neurons from operating normally, impairing cognition and causing emotional swings. Studies have indicated that acetaldehyde may be a factor in symptoms like irritation, difficulty concentrating, and brain fog.

Yeast overgrowth not only directly affects brain function but can also lead to vitamin deficiencies, which worsen mood disorders. Candida consumes sugars and carbs, which causes them to exhaust vital elements including zinc, magnesium, and B vitamins. The synthesis of neurotransmitters and healthy brain function depend on these nutrients. An insufficiency of these nutrients may result in weariness, irritability, and mood fluctuations.

It is crucial to comprehend the complex interaction between mental health and yeast overgrowth in order to create symptom management plans. Even while antifungal drugs and other medical treatments may be required to treat candidiasis, lifestyle changes and holistic methods are just as vital in promoting general health.

The most important thing is to eat a diet that promotes gut health. This entails cutting back on sugar and refined carbohydrates, which serve as yeast's main energy sources. Rather, concentrating on a whole foods diet full of healthy fats, lean proteins, and veggies can help to reduce symptoms and support a balanced gut microbiota. Foods high in probiotics, such as yoghurt and fermented veggies, can also assist to restore equilibrium in the stomach by introducing good bacteria.

Another essential component of treating mood disorders and yeast overgrowth is stress management. Prolonged stress has been demonstrated to have an effect on gut health and may be a factor in Candida overgrowth. Including methods for reducing stress, such yoga, meditation, and deep breathing exercises, can help control the body's reaction to stress and enhance mental health in general.

Regular exercise is essential for supporting a healthy gut and happy mood in addition to stress management. It has been demonstrated that engaging in physical activity supports a diverse gut flora and releases endorphins, which are organic mood enhancers. Including enjoyable activities in your routine might have positive effects on your mental and physical health.

It is crucial to address any underlying problems, such as hormone imbalances or immune system dysfunctions, in addition to these lifestyle changes. Identifying and treating these underlying reasons with the assistance of a healthcare professional who specialises in integrative medicine can offer a more thorough approach to treating the yeast overgrowth and any related mood disorders.

In conclusion, there is a complicated and nuanced relationship between yeast infections and mood disorders. Gaining knowledge about how yeast overgrowth affects mental health and putting symptom management techniques into practise can greatly enhance general wellbeing. People can take back control of their health and emotional and physical well-being by adopting holistic methods, stress management strategies, and lifestyle changes.

# Addressing Anxiety and Depression

It's common to underestimate the relationship between yeast infections and mental health. Nonetheless, a number of studies show that people with disorders such as Candida overgrowth are more likely to have elevated levels of anxiety and depression. This relationship can be explained by a number of things, such as the effect that an excess of pathogenic microorganisms has on the gut-brain axis and the inflammatory reaction that yeast infections cause. Moreover, the agony and humiliation brought on by yeast infections can cause severe psychological anguish, aggravating pre-existing anxiety and melancholy or even bringing them on in vulnerable people.

Understanding and resolving these psychological obstacles is essential to the whole management of yeast infections. It is critical to realise that addressing the physical symptoms on their own could offer brief respite. However, care for one's mental and emotional health is also necessary to promote long-term healing and wellness. Therefore, in order to assist people in navigating the nuanced relationship between yeast infections and mental health, I advise a holistic strategy that incorporates therapy techniques, dietary changes, and access to professional support resources.

The use of therapeutic approaches is essential in treating the anxiety and despair brought on by yeast infections. Cognitive-behavioral therapy (CBT) is one of the most successful modalities; it focuses on recognising and changing harmful thought patterns and behaviours. Through the development of useful coping skills, cognitive behavioural therapy (CBT) enables people to question illogical beliefs and swap them out for more adaptable and constructive ways of thinking. Patients can explore their emotional causes, create healthy coping strategies, and find emotional relief from yeast infections by working with a qualified therapist.

Furthermore, complementary and alternative methods can also be very helpful in treating depression and anxiety. Deep breathing exercises, yoga, and meditation have all been demonstrated to lower stress levels, encourage relaxation, and enhance mental health in general. These methods are simple to implement into everyday schedules, enabling people to develop resilience and serenity despite the difficulties caused by yeast infections. In addition, additional self-help methods like journaling, painting, and doing enjoyable things can support people in processing their feelings and taking back control of their lives.

Another important component of treating anxiety and sadness in the setting of yeast infections is changing one's lifestyle. Anxiety and depression can be directly improved and mental health elevated by leading a healthy lifestyle. Maintaining a balanced diet that promotes gut health and reduces inflammation is crucial, first and foremost. Eating foods high in probiotics, such yoghurt and fermented veggies, can help restore the gut flora and reduce the symptoms of anxiety and depression. Additionally, eliminating trigger foods—such as processed and sugary foods—can help stop the overgrowth of yeast and the ensuing mental health problems.

Apart from dietary adjustments, consistent physical activity has been demonstrated to be advantageous for psychological health. Natural mood enhancers called endorphins are released more frequently when one is physically active. Exercises like yoga, cycling, and brisk walking help increase mood, ease stress, and enhance mental health in general. In addition, getting enough sleep each night is crucial for emotional fortitude. A regular sleep schedule and a calm sleeping environment help people effectively manage the anxiety and despair brought on by yeast infections.

While self-help methods and lifestyle changes are important, getting professional help is frequently required for those who are experiencing severe depression and anxiety. Psychologists and psychiatrists are examples of mental health specialists who can create customised treatment regimens based on the individual needs of each patient. Individual and group therapy sessions give patients the chance to examine their feelings, pick up useful coping mechanisms, and interact in a kind and understanding setting. Medication may occasionally be recommended to treat metabolic imbalances and relieve incapacitating symptoms.

In conclusion, treating anxiety and sadness brought on by yeast infections is a crucial component of all-encompassing treatment for yeast infections. People can begin a holistic recovery journey that includes therapy methods, lifestyle changes, and professional support alternatives by realising the connection between mental health and physical well-being. By implementing these tactics, people can learn important lessons about taking care of their mental health and open the door to a better, more satisfying existence free from the hassles of yeast infections. Recall that healing involves feeding the mind and spirit in addition to treating the bodily ailments.

# The Gut-Brain Connection

As a physician and health and wellness coach, I've learned how profoundly our gut health affects our general wellbeing. In the realm of holistic healthcare, there has been an increasing interest in the complex and intriguing interaction known as the gut-brain axis, which exists between the gut and the brain.

Mental health can be significantly impacted by yeast infections, particularly those caused by Candida overgrowth. Together with other microbes, one kind of yeast that is normally present in our stomachs is called candida. Nevertheless, Candida can overgrow and result in a number of health issues, including yeast infections, when there is an imbalance in the gut flora.

A leaky gut is a disorder where the intestinal wall lining becomes more permeable, enabling toxins and harmful microbes to enter the circulation. This can be caused by an overgrowth of yeast. This may set off an inflammatory and immunological reaction that impacts the brain and exacerbates mental health conditions like sadness and anxiety.

Studies have demonstrated that the brain and the gut communicate in both directions. Neurotransmitters like serotonin—often referred to as the "feel-good" hormone—are produced in the gut. In actuality, the gut produces about 90% of serotonin. Emotional imbalances and mood disorders can result from dysbiosis of the gut, which can impact serotonin production.

Moreover, millions of bacteria reside in the gut and are essential to our general health. These bacteria in our stomach, referred to as the gut microbiota, aid in vitamin production, aid in food digestion, and guard against dangerous infections. An imbalance in the gut flora might cause problems with neurotransmitter production and mental health.

Thus, what steps can we take to strengthen the gut-brain axis and improve our gut health?

Diet and nutrition are two important tactics. Eating a diet high in complete, unprocessed foods helps lower inflammation and promote a healthy gut microbiome. Consuming meals high in fibre, such as fruits, vegetables, and whole grains, can support healthy digestion by nourishing the gut flora. Probiotics—good bacteria that support gut health—are another benefit of fermented foods like yoghurt, kefir, sauerkraut, and kimchi.

Stress management is another crucial component of intestinal health. The neurological system maintains a close connection between the gut and the brain, and long-term stress can negatively affect gut health. Better gut health and mental well-being can be supported by incorporating stress-reduction practises including mindfulness, meditation, deep breathing exercises, and regular physical activity.

Furthermore, controlling yeast infections and preserving gut health may benefit from avoiding or consuming fewer items that encourage yeast overgrowth. High-glycemic carbs, processed foods, alcohol, and refined sugars are some examples of these foods. Choosing complete, nutrient-dense foods and low-sugar substitutes can help establish an environment in the stomach that is less conducive to yeast overgrowth.

Supporting gut health can also be facilitated by supplements. Probiotics, which are living bacteria that boost immunity when ingested, can aid in reestablishing the proper balance of gut flora. On the other hand, prebiotics, a form of fibre found in foods like onions, garlic, artichokes, and bananas, nourish the good bacteria in the stomach. Furthermore, it has been demonstrated that some herbs and natural medicines, like grapefruit seed extract, garlic extract, and oregano oil, have antifungal qualities and can help treat yeast infections.

In summary, the gut-brain relationship is an intriguing field of research that emphasises the significance of preserving a healthy gut for our general wellbeing. We may enhance both our physical and mental well-being by realising the connection between gut health and emotional stability and by putting supportive measures in place for our digestive systems. We can develop a healthy balance that supports optimum health and energy by fostering the gut-brain connection.

# Building Resilience and Emotional Strength

I'll go into detail on developing emotional fortitude and perseverance in the face of yeast infections in this chapter. I'll go over some methods and approaches with you that will support you in developing a positive outlook and navigating the emotional rollercoaster that this illness frequently brings with it. By putting these habits into practise, you'll be more prepared to take on and successfully navigate the obstacles that lie ahead.

Understanding the value of holistic care is crucial as we set out on this path to develop emotional fortitude and resilience. Holistic healthcare treats your entire well-being, including your mental and emotional health, in addition to your physical ailments. Thus, when it comes to treating yeast infections, it is imperative to take a comprehensive strategy.

Empirical evidence indicates that emotional health is a critical component of the healing process. According to studies, people who have a resilient view and a positive mindset frequently recover more quickly from their treatments and have better results. By focusing on our mental well-being, we may give ourselves the assistance we need to recover from trauma.

The following are some methods that readers will learn for enhancing emotional fortitude and perseverance in the face of yeast infections:

1. Mindfulness and Meditation:

Mindfulness and meditation are two of the best strategies for developing emotional fortitude and resilience. These techniques entail developing an awareness and acceptance of the current moment as well as focusing your attention there. You can lower stress, enhance emotional stability, and increase resilience by practising mindfulness and meditation on a daily basis.

2. Positive Affirmations and Visualizations:

Resilience and emotional strength can be developed with the help of positive affirmations and visualisations. You may reprogram your brain to overcome negative thoughts and emotions and focus on the possibility of healing by repeating affirmations and visualising good results. By incorporating these routines into your daily life, you can develop emotional resilience and keep a positive view when faced with obstacles.

3. Seeking Support:

Seeking help from friends, family, or support groups is crucial because managing a yeast infection can be emotionally taxing. It can be relieving and validating to share your feelings, worries, and experiences with like-minded people. You may provide each other support, direction, and courage as you go through the highs and lows of this journey together.

4. Self-Care:

Consistent self-care is necessary to keep emotional stability and build resilience. This can include things like exercising frequently, getting enough sleep, eating a healthy diet, practising relaxation techniques, and engaging in enjoyable and gratifying hobbies. Taking care of your physical and emotional needs is essential to maintaining a good outlook and overcoming the challenges posed by a yeast infection.

5. Journaling:

Maintaining a journal can be an effective strategy for managing emotions, lowering stress levels, and developing resilience. Putting your ideas and emotions down on paper helps you make sense of your experiences and obtain perspective. Furthermore, journaling gives you a way to express yourself and let go of suppressed feelings. You can strengthen your emotional resilience and gain a better knowledge of your feelings by keeping a journal on a regular basis.

6. Goal Setting:

Having a positive mindset and developing resilience can be facilitated by setting goals. You can feel motivated and accomplished when you manage your yeast infection by creating modest, manageable goals and tracking your progress. You can become more emotionally resilient and strong in the long run by using this technique to help you remain proactive and focused on your healing process.

7. Cognitive Restructuring:

Cognitive restructuring is the process of recognising, questioning, and substituting more realistic, positive ideas for negative ones. You can increase your resilience and cultivate a more optimistic view by changing the way you think and feel about your yeast infection and putting more emphasis on possible remedies and positive results. This method gives you the ability to master your ideas and feelings, enabling you to take on obstacles head-on.

By using these strategies, readers can manage yeast infections and develop emotional fortitude and resilience. You can deal with the difficulties of this illness more skillfully and gracefully by promoting psychological well-being and keeping an optimistic mindset. Recall that developing resilience is a lifelong process that calls for consistent practise and commitment. However, you may build the emotional fortitude required to get past any challenge you face with commitment and persistence.

We shall examine the connection between food and yeast infections in the upcoming chapter. You will learn how some foods can exacerbate yeast overgrowth and how making dietary changes can help you on your path to recovery. Now let's explore the realm of nutrition and equip ourselves with the skills and information needed to properly treat yeast infections.

# Chapter 14: Yeast Infections and Skin Health

# Yeast Infections and Skin Conditions

Yeast infections, or candidiasis, are caused by an overabundance of the fungus Candida within the body. Although the body naturally contains small amounts of Candida, a number of circumstances can upset the delicate balance and cause an overgrowth. A compromised immune system is one of these factors, and it can be brought on by a number of things, such as chronic illnesses, stress, poor food, and sleep deprivation.

The immune system's ability to control the population of Candida is diminished when it is weakened. Consequently, the fungus have the ability to proliferate and disperse, impacting various bodily parts, including the skin. The skin serves as a barrier to keep out external infections, but it can also cause a variety of skin diseases if the balance of microorganisms on the skin is upset.

The appearance of rashes is a typical cutaneous symptom of yeast infections. The look of these rashes might vary, showing either as bigger, raised regions or as tiny red pimples. In addition, they could be accompanied by discomfort, burning, and itching. A person's quality of life may be greatly impacted by these symptoms, which can include irritation, poor productivity, and sleep difficulties.

Yeast infections can also result in excruciating itching in addition to rashes. The itch may originate in one spot on the body or go across it. It can be quite distressing for people to have continual itching, which makes it difficult for them to focus on daily activities and causes severe discomfort and aggravation.

Inflammation is another typical sign of yeast infections on the skin. Inflammation results from the body's immune system being activated due to Candida overgrowth. In the affected locations, this inflammation may result in redness, swelling, and pain. In extreme circumstances, blisters or ulcerations filled with pus may even result.

Effective management and treatment of various skin disorders depend on an understanding of the relationship between yeast infections and these conditions. We can lessen the symptoms and stop yeast infections from coming again by treating the overgrowth's underlying cause.

Boosting immunity is one of the first stages in treating yeast infections and related skin disorders. This can be accomplished by making lifestyle changes such as eating a well-balanced, nutrient-dense diet, exercising frequently, practising stress reduction, and getting enough sleep. Probiotics, garlic, and oregano oil are a few other herbs and supplements that can boost immunity and encourage a balanced population of microorganisms in the body.

Addressing any underlying issues that might be causing the immune system to weaken is also crucial. This could entail treating any underlying medical illnesses like diabetes or autoimmune disorders, recognising and resolving the causes of ongoing stress, and making nutritional improvements.

Keeping up with hygiene is also crucial for treating skin disorders and yeast infections. Preventing further irritation can be achieved by cleaning the afflicted areas with mild, pH-balanced cleansers and avoiding harsh soaps or perfumed products. Wearing breathable, loose-fitting clothing and avoiding prolonged wetness in the affected regions can also help promote healing and stop the infection from spreading.

Topical antifungal drugs may be recommended in situations where lifestyle adjustments are ineffective or the symptoms are severe. These drugs function by preventing Candida from growing and by lessening the swelling and irritation brought on by yeast infections. But it's crucial to take these drugs under a doctor's supervision, as using them incorrectly or excessively might cause resistance and worsen existing skin issues.

In conclusion, yeast infections can cause rashes, itching, and inflammation, all of which can have a significant effect on a person's skin health. Effective management and treatment of various skin disorders depend on an understanding of the relationship between yeast infections and these conditions. People can effectively treat and prevent yeast infections on the skin by taking care of the underlying causes, boosting the immune system, and practising good hygiene. By using a holistic approach to healthcare, I hope to give people all-encompassing solutions to support their general well-being and skin health.

# Skin Care Tips for Yeast Infection Management

The affected areas of yeast infections can become swollen, itchy, and irritated. If not handled appropriately, this can cause discomfort and even more issues. To relieve symptoms and promote healing, it is crucial to follow a mild, hydrating skin care regimen that also incorporates the use of natural therapies.

Gentle washing is one of the first steps in treating yeast infections. To prevent more aggravation, it's critical to handle the affected regions with caution. I advise using a soft cleanser made especially for sensitive skin types or a moderate, fragrance-free soap. Harsh soaps and cleansers with fragrances or other unpleasant ingredients can upset the skin's natural pH balance and exacerbate yeast infection symptoms. You may efficiently eliminate pollutants without endangering the skin further by using a mild cleanser.

It's critical to completely dry the impacted areas after cleaning. Keeping the skin dry is crucial to controlling and avoiding yeast infections because moisture creates the perfect habitat for yeast to flourish in. Instead of rubbing, I advise gently patting the skin dry with a fresh towel because friction irritates the skin even more. To guarantee thorough drying, it could also be helpful to use a hairdryer on a low, cool setting, especially in areas of the skin where moisture tends to collect.

Moisturizing the skin becomes essential for treating yeast infections once it has grown dry. Moisturizers can aid in healing, itch relief, and skin calming. To prevent escalating the illness, it's crucial to select the appropriate moisturiser. Seek for hypoallergenic and fragrance-free goods; these are less prone to irritate skin. Furthermore, choose moisturisers with moisturising components like glycerin, hyaluronic acid, or ceramides, as these support the preservation and restoration of the skin's natural moisture barrier.

Natural treatments may occasionally offer extra comfort and assistance in the management of yeast infections. For instance, the antifungal qualities of tea tree oil can aid in the fight against yeast overgrowth. Tea tree oil can be unpleasant if used topically, so it's important to dilute it before putting it on skin. One teaspoon of carrier oil (such coconut or olive oil) to five drops of tea tree oil is an acceptable dilution ratio. After applying this combination to the afflicted areas, rinse it off after about 15 minutes. Twice daily, repeat this procedure until the symptoms subside.

Apple cider vinegar is another possible efficient natural treatment. Yeast cannot grow in the acidic environment that apple cider vinegar produces. To prevent additional skin irritation, it is crucial to dilute apple cider vinegar before applying it topically. Apply a solution made from one cup water and one tablespoon apple cider vinegar to the afflicted regions using a clean cotton ball. Before rinsing off, let it sit for a few minutes. You can repeat this once or twice a day until the symptoms go away.

Although these home remedies may offer some relief, it's important to keep in mind that they should be taken in addition to medical care. Before starting any new treatment regimen, speak with your doctor, particularly if you have sensitive skin or are prone to adverse reactions.

It's critical to address any underlying issues that might be causing recurrent yeast infections in addition to following these skin care recommendations. This could entail adjusting one's diet, practising stress management, and changing one's way of life. Managing yeast infections holistically can result in long-term alleviation and enhanced general health.

In summary, taking good care of your skin is essential to controlling yeast infections. Readers can easily ease symptoms and help the healing process by implementing natural therapies, moisturising tactics, and mild cleansing practises. To find the best course of action for specific requirements and to address any underlying causes that might be causing recurring yeast infections, it is crucial to speak with a healthcare provider. People can treat their yeast infection and experience long-lasting relief with a thorough strategy and regular skin care regimen.

# Preventive Measures for Skin Health

The cornerstone to avoiding yeast infections and preserving skin health is good cleanliness. Since the skin is our body's first line of protection against dangerous microorganisms, it is crucial to keep it clean and in good condition. I counsel my patients to start a regular skincare regimen that entails washing their skin gently with a cleanser free of sulphates or mild soap. Tough soaps have the ability to deplete the skin of its natural oils, making it parched and prone to illness. Excessive scrubbing should also be avoided since this might damage the skin's protective layer and cause trauma.

It's essential to hydrate the skin after cleansing in order to preserve its natural barrier and replenish moisture. Seek for moisturisers that are free of harsh chemicals and scents, and that are tailored to your specific skin type. Hydrating your skin is an easy way to prevent infections because dry skin is more likely to get them.

Clothes selection is a crucial component of preventive skin care. Nylon and polyester are examples of synthetic materials that retain heat and moisture, which makes yeast growth optimal. Rather, use natural textiles that allow for air circulation, such as linen and cotton, to keep the skin cool and dry. Skin breakouts can also result from friction and discomfort caused by tight clothing. Pick loose-fitting clothing that won't press against your skin whenever you can.

I constantly stress to my patients the significance of staying away from irritants that can weaken the integrity of their skin and increase their vulnerability to infections. Some skincare products, laundry detergents, and fabric softeners include harsh chemicals that can irritate skin and upset the delicate balance of the skin's microflora. It's critical to read product labels and select hypoallergenic, mild, and irritant-free products that don't include artificial perfumes or alcohol.

It's also critical to consider how our lifestyle decisions affect the health of our skin. For example, smoking deteriorates not just our general health but also the skin's capacity to repair itself and fend against pathogens. According to research, smoking can weaken the skin's defences against infections, which can lead to a variety of skin disorders. Without a doubt, one of the best things we can do for the health of our skin is to stop smoking.

Our entire health, including the condition of our skin, is greatly influenced by the food we eat. Eating a nutritious, vitamin- and antioxidant-rich, well-balanced diet can strengthen the skin's barrier function and strengthen the immune system. Eating a diet rich in fruits, vegetables, whole grains, and lean proteins will help supply the building blocks needed for good skin. It's also critical to limit your intake of processed and sugary meals because they can upset the delicate balance of your skin's microbiota and promote yeast overgrowth.

Sustaining healthy skin requires not just a balanced diet but also drinking enough water. The body needs water to function at its best, and being dehydrated can cause dry, cracked skin that is more prone to infections. Try to consume eight glasses or more of water each day, and drink more when you're exercising more or it's hot outside.

Stress has been shown to have a substantial effect on our skin as well as our general health. Excessive stress can impair immunological function, reducing its ability to fend off infections. Thus, integrating stress-reduction strategies into our everyday lives is essential to preserving the health of our skin. This can involve relaxing pursuits like yoga, deep breathing techniques, meditation, or engaging in hobbies. Skin infections can be greatly avoided by making emotional health a priority and setting aside time for self-care.

Finally, it's critical to consider the possible negative effects of specific medications and how they may affect the condition of your skin. Antibiotics, for instance, have been shown to upset the microflora's normal equilibrium on the skin, increasing the likelihood of yeast overgrowth. It's crucial to talk to your doctor about precautions you may take to reduce your risk of yeast infections if you're taking antibiotics. Probiotics and other supplements that maintain a balanced microbiota may fall under this category.

In summary, preserving skin health and averting yeast infections necessitates a comprehensive strategy that includes good hygiene, attire selection, and averting irritants. We may create an environment where our skin is less vulnerable to infections by using proper hygiene practises, dressing appropriately, and being aware of potential irritants. We can further promote the general health of our skin by embracing a healthy lifestyle that includes stress management, a balanced diet, enough hydration, and knowledge of the adverse effects of medications. By taking these precautionary steps, we may clear the way for thorough control of yeast infections and have happier, healthier skin.

# Treating Skin Complications of Yeast Infections

Dear readers,

We will examine the many approaches to treating skin problems brought on by yeast infections in this chapter. These issues can be very upsetting because they hurt and affect our general wellbeing. But with the correct information and resources, we can deal with these problems and get rid of the symptoms.

As a physician and supporter of holistic medicine, I think that treating yeast infections and related skin issues should be approached holistically. This entails treating the underlying causes in addition to treating the symptoms and advancing general health and fitness.

1. Understanding Skin Complications:

It is important to comprehend the many kinds of skin issues that might result from yeast infections before moving on to treatment choices. Yeast infections can cause symptoms including redness, itching, rash, and pain in the skin, among other parts of the body.

Common skin complications associated with yeast infections include:

- Cutaneous Candidiasis: This ailment appears as a red, itchy rash that typically appears in warm, damp body parts like the skin's folds or in between the toes.

- Intertrigo: When there is wetness and friction in places where the skin folds, such the groyne, beneath the breasts, or under the armpits, it can cause intertrigo. It may result in rash, redness, and even excruciating sores.

- Diaper rash: Diaper rash associated to yeast infection is more common in infants and early children and is characterised by redness, itching, and little red bumps.

Understanding the specific skin complication you are experiencing is crucial for choosing the most appropriate treatment.

2. Treatment Options:

a) Topical Creams:

Topical antifungal creams are one of the most widely used therapy choices for skin issues resulting from yeast infections. The active components in these lotions assist to directly target the proliferation of yeast and alleviate symptoms.

It is imperative that you select a topical cream that is meant to treat yeast infections. Seek for creams that contain nystatin, miconazole, or clotrimazole, among other antifungal medications. Following the directions on the package, apply the cream to the affected region, making sure to cover the whole area.

b) Antifungal Medications:

Sometimes oral antifungal drugs are administered, particularly if the skin issues are severe or extensive. These drugs target the excess of yeast throughout the body systemically, and they can be quite helpful in treating severe skin problems.

A healthcare provider should be consulted before beginning any oral antifungal drug. When deciding on the best drug and dose, they will consider a number of things, including your medical history and unique ailment.

c) Soothing Remedies:

Apart from pharmaceutical interventions, there exist many analgesic cures that can mitigate the discomfort correlated with skin issues resulting from yeast infections. For milder situations, these therapies can be taken alone or in conjunction with other medical treatments.

- Warm Water Soaks: The irritated area can be made to feel less red and itchy by soaking it in warm water infused with Epsom salts.

- Natural Oils: The skin can be soothed and symptoms reduced by using natural oils to the affected area, such as coconut oil, tea tree oil, or lavender oil. Patch testing these oils beforehand is crucial to make sure you don't experience an allergic reaction.

- Cool Compresses: Temporary relief can be achieved by applying a cool, damp compress or cloth to the affected area, which can help reduce irritation.

d) Lifestyle Modifications:

In order to aid in the healing process, some lifestyle adjustments are also necessary while treating yeast infection-related skin problems. Here are some crucial pointers:

- Keep the affected area clean and dry: Because warmth and moisture can make yeast infections worse, it's critical to keep the affected region dry and clean. Instead of dressing too tight, use airy, loose fabrics.

- Practice good hygiene: Maintaining good cleanliness is essential to controlling and avoiding yeast infections. Make sure you use a mild, fragrance-free soap to wash the affected region, and pat dry rather than rubbing.

- Avoid irritants: Some products can aggravate yeast infections and irritate the skin, such as scented soaps, douches, and feminine hygiene products. It is best to stay away from these goods and use kinder substitutes.

- Maintain a healthy diet: Your body can fight off yeast infections and boost its immune system with a well-balanced, nutrient-rich diet. Consume foods high in probiotics, such yoghurt, to help maintain a balanced population of good bacteria in your body.

You can encourage long-term recovery and enhance the efficacy of the treatment choices by putting these lifestyle changes into practise.

Conclusion:

You can control yeast infection-related skin concerns and alleviate discomfort by learning about the many treatment options available and implementing a holistic strategy. Whether you choose to use topical creams, antifungal drugs, soothing therapies, or alter your lifestyle, it's critical to customise your strategy to your unique condition and consult a healthcare provider.

Recall that treating yeast infection-related skin problems takes time and effort. You will eventually feel better and recover control over your health and well-being if you stick to your treatment plan.

We will discuss ways to keep your body in a healthy balance and prevent yeast infections in the upcoming chapter to reduce the likelihood of a recurrence.

Until then, remember to prioritise your health and take care of yourself.

With love and well wishes,

Dr. Ankita Kashyap

# Chapter 15: Yeast Infections and Immune System

# Understanding the Immune System and Yeast Infections

It's critical to explore the complexities of our body's defensive mechanism in order to fully understand the relationship between yeast infections and the immune system. To defend our bodies from dangerous pathogens like bacteria, viruses, and fungus, the immune system is a sophisticated network of cells, tissues, and organs. Its fundamental objective is to preserve our bodies' health and homeostasis.

Leukocytes, another name for white blood cells, are important components of the immune system. The innate immune system and the adaptive immune system are the two primary groups of these cells. The adaptive immune system is specially designed to target and eradicate particular diseases that the body has already encountered, whereas the innate immune system serves as the body's first line of defence and a quick reaction system.

The immune system is essential for stopping yeast overgrowth and recurrence in cases of yeast infections. The most prevalent kind of yeast, Candida, is found naturally in human bodies. On the other hand, an overgrowth can happen and lead to a yeast infection if the immune system and yeast are not in equilibrium.

A compromised immune system is one of the primary variables that can affect the immune system's capacity to regulate yeast overgrowth. The immune system can be weakened by a number of things, such as long-term stress, poor eating habits, sleep deprivation, and underlying medical disorders like diabetes or HIV/AIDS. Yeast infections are more likely when the immune system is compromised because it is less able to control the body's yeast levels.

In addition to being involved in the regulation of yeast development, the immune system may also be adversely affected by yeast overgrowth. An immunological response may be triggered by an overabundance of yeast in the body, which can cause inflammation. The immune system may subsequently be further compromised by this ongoing inflammation, leading to a vicious cycle of immunological dysregulation and yeast overgrowth.

According to research, those with weakened immune systems—such as those with HIV/AIDS or undergoing chemotherapy—are more prone to get yeast infections again. Furthermore, research has shown that people with compromised immune systems find it more challenging to treat yeast infections than people with strong immune systems.

Considering that yeast infections and the immune system are mutually exclusive, maintaining and avoiding yeast overgrowth requires immune system assistance. Strategies that fortify the immune system and aid in preserving a healthy equilibrium between it and the yeast in our bodies should be part of a comprehensive approach to managing yeast infections.

Changes in lifestyle are essential to improve immunological health. Sustaining immunological function, for instance, requires adequate nourishment. A diet high in fruits, vegetables, whole grains, lean protein, and healthy fats gives the immune system the nourishment it needs to perform at its best. Through proper nutrition, we may strengthen our immune system and improve its capacity to fight yeast overgrowth.

Another important component of immunological health is stress management. Prolonged stress can significantly affect the immune system, making it less effective in its job. Including stress-relieving practises like yoga, meditation, or deep breathing exercises can help the immune system regain equilibrium and lower the chance of yeast overgrowth.

Even more, a healthy immune system depends on getting enough sleep. The body heals and renews itself when we sleep, and the immune system is no exception. The immune system can become weakened by inadequate or poor sleep, leaving the body more vulnerable to infections, including yeast infections. Through the practise of good sleep hygiene and getting adequate restorative sleep every night, we can strengthen our immune system's defences against yeast overgrowth.

Apart from alterations in lifestyle, a range of self-care methods can also be beneficial in bolstering immune function and controlling yeast infections. These could be things like maintaining good cleanliness, getting regular exercise, and include immune-stimulating vitamins and herbs in our diets. Studies have indicated that some supplements, such garlic, probiotics, vitamin C, and vitamin D, can boost immunity and lower the risk of yeast infections.

Ultimately, immunity depends on preserving psychological well-being. Negative emotions and psychological stress, including despair or worry, can impair immunity and raise the possibility of yeast overgrowth. We can address the emotional and psychological variables that effect immunological health and get better results by integrating psychology-related treatments and counselling into our comprehensive approach to managing yeast infections.

To sum up, in order to effectively prevent and treat yeast overgrowth, it is critical to comprehend the immune system's involvement in managing yeast infections. The immune system and yeast are in a delicate balance, and we can support immunological health and prevent yeast infections by making lifestyle alterations, practising self-care, and maintaining psychological well-being. Recall that the immune system is an effective weapon in our body's battle against yeast overgrowth, and that we can become experts at treating yeast infections if we have the correct information and resources.

# Lifestyle Modifications for Immune Support

Dietary Changes:

Dietary adjustments are among the most significant lifestyle changes you can make to boost your immune system. Eating a nutritious, well-balanced diet that gives your body the vitamins, minerals, and antioxidants it needs to fend against illnesses is essential. Including foods that are recognised to strengthen the immune system will significantly increase your resistance against yeast infections.

For example, increasing the amount of fruits and vegetables in your diet can supply you with a variety of vital nutrients. Vitamin C-rich foods include bell peppers, citrus fruits, and berries. These foods can also increase the formation of white blood cells, which are important components of your immune system's defence mechanism.

Foods high in probiotics ought to be a mainstay of your diet as well. Probiotics play a critical role in preserving the delicate balance of bacteria in your digestive system, which inhibits the formation of yeast. Probiotics from fermented foods, such as kefir, kimchi, sauerkraut, and yoghurt, are great for boosting immunity and preventing yeast infections.

Limiting or avoiding specific foods that can weaken your immune system and raise your chance of developing yeast infections is just as crucial. Refined carbs and sugar, found in processed snacks, sugar-filled drinks, and white bread, can feed the yeast and encourage its overgrowth. Limiting alcohol and caffeine intake is also recommended because they can impair immunity.

Exercise:

Engaging in regular physical activity is crucial not only for preserving a healthy weight but also for enhancing immunological function. Moderate-intensity exercises, like brisk walking, cycling, or swimming, can help your body's immune cells circulate more freely and fight off infections more effectively.

In addition, exercise lowers stress, which is essential for boosting immunity. Prolonged stress can impair immunity, increasing your vulnerability to diseases such as yeast infections. You may boost your immune system's reaction, reduce stress, and enhance your mental health by making regular exercise a part of your routine.

Stress Reduction Techniques:

To boost your immune system and lower your risk of yeast infections, you can incorporate a variety of stress-reduction tactics into your daily routine in addition to exercising. Prolonged stress can impair immune system function, which facilitates the spread of diseases.

Reducing stress and fostering calm can be achieved by engaging in relaxation practises including yoga, meditation, and deep breathing exercises. It has been demonstrated that using these methods will increase the relaxation response, which will offset the effects of stress hormones.

Additionally, you can significantly lower your stress levels by partaking in enjoyable and relaxing activities. Making time for hobbies, enjoying the great outdoors, or spending time with close friends and family are all excellent ways to boost your immune system and general well-being.

Sleep:

When it comes to immunological support, getting enough sleep is sometimes overlooked. Your body, especially your immune system, repairs and rejuvenates itself as you sleep. Your immune system might be weakened by sleep deprivation, leaving you more vulnerable to infections, including yeast infections.

A regular sleep schedule is essential for promoting both longer and higher-quality slumber. Aim for seven to nine hours of undisturbed sleep per night, and make sure the room is dark, quiet, and at a comfortable temperature to promote healthy sleep.

If you have trouble falling asleep, you can help yourself sleep better by using relaxation techniques before bed. Some of these strategies include reading a book, having a warm bath, or practising mindfulness.

Coping Strategies:

Lastly, in order to control stress and keep it from impairing your immune system, it is essential to establish healthy coping mechanisms. Finding healthy and adaptable coping mechanisms for stress is crucial because prolonged stress can compromise immunity and raise the risk of yeast infections.

Seeking support from dependable friends or family members, self-care practises that encourage relaxation and well-being, such taking a warm bath, pursuing interests or creative outlets, and getting regular exercise are some coping mechanisms that you could find useful.

Incorporating stress-reduction strategies like journaling, deep breathing exercises, and mindfulness can also provide you a sense of control and resilience while you deal with difficult circumstances.

In conclusion, you may dramatically lower your risk of developing yeast infections and preserve a healthy balance in your body by implementing lifestyle changes that emphasise strengthening your immune system and lowering stress. A holistic strategy to managing yeast infections must include dietary adjustments, regular exercise, stress reduction practises, sleep prioritisation, and the development of appropriate coping mechanisms. You will receive further information and approaches in the upcoming chapters to help you master the treatment of yeast infections and attain optimal health.

# Immune-Boosting Supplements and Herbs

As a medical expert who supports holistic approaches to wellness, I firmly think that the immune system has the ability to fend against illnesses and preserve general health. A robust immune system is especially important while dealing with yeast infections since it can aid in preventing the overabundance of yeast in the body. I will go into the realm of immune-stimulating vitamins and herbs that may help with the treatment of yeast infections in this subchapter. I'll go over their possible advantages, usage restrictions, and possible interactions.

1. Vitamin C:

Strong antioxidants like vitamin C are essential for boosting the immune system. It aids in promoting white blood cell formation, which is necessary for warding off infections, including yeast infections. Moreover, vitamin C promotes the synthesis of collagen, a protein that improves the tensile strength and integrity of various tissues, including the skin and mucous membranes, all of which are susceptible to yeast infections.

For immunological support, I usually advise taking 1000–2000 mg of vitamin C daily. It's crucial to remember that consuming too much vitamin C can result in diarrhoea. Before including any supplements in your routine, it is always advisable to speak with a healthcare provider, particularly if you are taking any drugs.

2. Vitamin D:

In addition to its well-known effects on calcium absorption and bone health, vitamin D is essential for immune system performance. Studies have demonstrated that vitamin D lowers the risk of infections by regulating the immune response. Yeast infections are more likely to occur in those with low vitamin D levels.

For immunological support, I usually suggest 1000–2000 IU of vitamin D3 daily. However, before beginning any supplementation, it is imperative to get your vitamin D levels checked. This will assist in figuring out the right dosage for you, as every person has different demands.

3. Zinc:

One mineral that is essential to immunological function is zinc. It promotes immunological responses and plays a role in the development and operation of immune cells. Additionally, zinc promotes wound healing, which is advantageous when yeast infections have damaged the skin and mucous membranes.

I normally give 30–50 mg of zinc per day for immune support. It is crucial to remember that consuming too much zinc might have negative consequences and interfere with the absorption of other minerals like copper. Seeking advice from a medical expert is recommended prior to beginning zinc supplements.

4. Echinacea:

Popular herb echinacea is well-known for strengthening the immune system. It has long been used to treat and prevent respiratory diseases such as the flu and colds. It is thought that echinacea improves immune function by promoting the generation and activation of immunological cells. It might be helpful in managing yeast infections since it might have antifungal qualities as well.

There are several ways to consume echinacea, such as teas, tinctures, and capsules. The type and concentration may affect the suggested dosage. For advice on proper usage, it is best to refer to the manufacturer's instructions or speak with a healthcare provider.

5. Garlic:

Strong-smelling garlic is an essential ingredient in many recipes and has a lot of health advantages. Because of its antibacterial and immune-stimulating qualities, it has been utilised for millennia. Allicin, a substance found in garlic, has been demonstrated to have antifungal qualities and may be useful in the treatment of yeast infections.

Garlic can be included in the diet, but it's also possible to purchase supplements in the form of tablets or capsules. It is crucial to remember that consuming too much garlic can irritate your stomach and interact with some drugs, such as blood thinners. It is advised to speak with a healthcare provider before starting any supplementation.

6. Probiotics:

Beneficial bacteria called probiotics are found in our stomachs by nature and are essential for a strong immune system. They guard against the proliferation of dangerous bacteria and yeast, such Candida, and aid in preserving the delicate balance of microorganisms in the gut. Probiotic supplements can assist in managing yeast infections and reestablishing the equilibrium of the gut microbiome.

Look for a probiotic supplement that has a range of strains, such as Bifidobacterium and Lactobacillus. For immune support, I often suggest a daily intake of 10–20 billion CFUs (colony-forming units). It is crucial to remember that every person has different needs, therefore for tailored advice, it is better to speak with a healthcare provider.

Conclusion:

Including immune-stimulating herbs and vitamins in your management strategy for yeast infections will help strengthen your defences against infection. Among the numerous alternatives are probiotics, zinc, echinacea, cloves, vitamin C, and vitamin D. But it's crucial to keep in mind that supplements cannot replace a healthy lifestyle that includes a balanced diet, consistent exercise, stress reduction, and enough sleep. As usual, it is best to speak with a healthcare provider before beginning any new supplement regimen, particularly if you are taking any drugs that may interfere with these supplements or have any underlying medical concerns. By working together, we can overcome the difficulties associated with managing yeast infections and set off on a path towards holistic wellbeing.

# Integrating Immune Support Into Daily Routine

When it comes to protecting your body from dangerous pathogens like bacteria, viruses, and fungus, the immune system is essential. Regarding yeast infections, the main cause of these illnesses is an overabundance of yeast in your body, which may be avoided with a strong immune system. Through the incorporation of straightforward yet effective tactics into your everyday routine, you may fortify your immune system and guarantee its optimal operation.

Including foods that boost the immune system in your diet is a great approach to strengthen your body's defences against illness. Your immune system can benefit from the vital elements it requires to function well if you eat a balanced diet high in vitamins, minerals, and antioxidants. Choose a range of vibrant fruits and vegetables, including leafy greens, cruciferous veggies like broccoli and cauliflower, citrus fruits, and berries. Vitamins that strengthen the immune system, including C and A, are abundant in these meals. In order to sustain energy and boost immunity, you should also include lean proteins, whole grains, and healthy fats like the omega-3 fatty acids found in fish and nuts.

In addition to concentrating on particular items, it's critical to consider the general calibre of your diet. Processed foods, sugary snacks, and excessive alcohol consumption should be avoided or minimised. These may impair your immunity and increase your vulnerability to infections, including yeast infections. Rather, make a deliberate effort to eat complete, nutrient-dense foods that will strengthen and hydrate your immune system and support its ideal operation.

Apart from maintaining a nutritious diet, a regular exercise regimen can make a big difference in immunological support.

Increasing blood circulation through physical exercise aids in the delivery of vital nutrients and oxygen to every area of your body, including the immune system. Frequent exercise also encourages the release of feel-good hormones called endorphins, which can lower stress and improve general wellbeing. On most days of the week, try to get in at least 30 minutes of moderate-intensity activity, such jogging, cycling, swimming, or brisk walking. Strength training activities can also aid in increasing muscle mass and bolstering the immune system.

Making stress reduction and relaxation a priority can also be extremely important for boosting your immune system. Prolonged stress might impair your immune system and increase your vulnerability to illnesses. Including stress-reduction strategies in your regular routine can boost your immune system and greatly enhance your general well-being. Techniques like yoga, tai chi, meditation, deep breathing, and mindfulness can lower stress, increase calm, and strengthen the immune system.

Sleep is a vital part of a healthy lifestyle, but it is sometimes disregarded when it comes to immune support. Your immune system must work properly for you to get enough good sleep. Your body, especially the immune system, heals and regenerates itself as you sleep. Sleep deprivation can impair immunity and raise the risk of infection. Prioritize creating a regular sleep schedule and strive for seven to nine hours of unbroken sleep each night. Maintain a peaceful, dark, and pleasant sleeping temperature in your bedroom to create a sleep-friendly atmosphere. Avoid using electronics right before bed since the blue light they create can disrupt your sleep cycle.

Adding vitamins to your diet will help strengthen your immune system even more. Even though eating whole meals is the best way to get all the nutrients you need, there are supplements that can help fill in any nutritional gaps and boost immunity. To find the right supplements for your unique requirements, speak with a qualified dietician or healthcare provider. Supplements that support the immune system that are frequently advised include probiotics, zinc, vitamin C, and vitamin D. It's crucial to remember that supplements should never take the place of a balanced diet and way of life; rather, they should enhance them.

Keeping the gut microbiota in good condition is another essential component of immune support. Bacteria are among the many types of microorganisms that live in the gut and are important for immunological function. A disruption in the balance of these microbiota can weaken immunity and raise the risk of infections, including yeast infections. Consuming foods high in probiotics, such as kefir, kimchi, sauerkraut, and yoghurt, can help your immune system and foster a healthy gut microbiota. A balanced gut flora can also be maintained by reducing the intake of processed meals, added sugars, and artificial sweeteners.

Finally, it's critical to take into account lifestyle and environmental factors that could affect your immune system. Steer clear of dangerous chemicals, pollutants, and toxins that might impair your immune system. Make thoughtful decisions to lessen your exposure to chemicals in the environment, like choosing natural personal care and cleaning supplies. Make a good work-life balance a priority as well by making time each day for self-care and relaxation. Take pauses, develop hobbies, spend time with loved ones, and schedule enjoyable and stress-relieving activities.

To sum up, incorporating immune support techniques into your daily routine is an effective approach to promote general wellbeing and reduce your chance of developing yeast infections. You can empower your immune system to work at its best by feeding it immune-supportive foods, exercising frequently, controlling stress, giving sleep priority, taking supplements, keeping your gut bacteria healthy, and being aware of your surroundings and lifestyle choices. Recall that consistency is essential and that these tactics complement one another. Your immune system will appreciate you for embracing them as a part of your lifestyle by defending you against infections and fostering long-term health and wellbeing.

# Chapter 16: Yeast Infections and Hormonal Health

# Hormonal Changes and Yeast Infections

The body naturally experiences changes in hormone levels, which are important for many physiological functions, including the menstrual cycle. These variations may have an impact on the interior milieu of the body, causing an imbalance that could lead to the emergence of yeast infections.

We must examine the complex mechanisms underlying the menstrual cycle in order to comprehend this relationship. Hormones, mainly progesterone and oestrogen, control the menstrual cycle. Together, these hormones help the body get ready for a possible pregnancy. However, these hormones' amounts vary during the cycle, impacting the vaginal environment at different times.

Estrogen levels rise during the follicular phase, which takes place in the first half of the menstrual cycle. In order to prepare for implantation, this hormone encourages the growth of the endometrium, or uterine lining. In addition, oestrogen has the ability to promote the growth of yeast, specifically Candida albicans. Although this type of yeast is frequently found in the vaginal environment, an overgrowth of it can result in a yeast infection.

Conversely, progesterone levels increase during the luteal phase, which takes place in the second half of the menstrual cycle. Progesterone promotes the growth of the uterine lining and gets the uterus ready for a possible pregnancy. Higher progesterone levels, though, may potentially be a factor in yeast overgrowth. It has been discovered that progesterone raises the amount of glycogen in the vaginal epithelium, which gives yeast development fuel.

It is important to understand that yeast infections are not directly caused by hormonal changes alone. Instead, they foster an atmosphere that is more favourable to the expansion of yeast. A number of variables, such as variations in the pH of the vagina, modifications in

204

the immune system, and the existence of other risk factors, may be involved.

For example, variations in progesterone and oestrogen levels might impact the pH of the vagina. The pH of the vagina is normally somewhat acidic, which inhibits the growth of dangerous bacteria and yeast. But as oestrogen levels rise in the follicular period, the pH shifts to an alkaline state, which is more conducive to yeast development. Similar to this, high progesterone levels during the luteal phase can cause a more alkaline pH, which encourages yeast overgrowth.

Hormonal changes can impact not only the pH of the vagina but also the body's immunological response. In order to control the growth of yeast and other microbes, the immune system is essential. Hormonal changes, however, have the potential to impair immunity and increase susceptibility to infections. This compromised immune response may facilitate the growth and overabundance of yeast.

In addition, it's critical to take into account any additional risk factors that can coexist with hormonal fluctuations. For instance, yeast infections are more common in those with weakened immune systems, such as those with diabetes or HIV. Similarly, using scented hygiene products or dressing in tight-fitting clothing are two lifestyle choices that might lead to yeast overgrowth.

An all-encompassing strategy is needed to manage yeast infections in the setting of hormonal fluctuations. Although treating the hormone changes directly might not be feasible or required, there are a number of tactics that can be used to manage and prevent yeast infections.

Keeping your vagina clean is essential for controlling yeast infections and hormonal fluctuations. Using strong soaps or douches is one way to do this, as they can upset the delicate balance of the vaginal environment. Instead, they ought to use mild, fragrance-free cleaning products and often wash with water.

Furthermore, breathable materials and loose-fitting apparel can aid in minimising moisture retention and enhancing vaginal ventilation. This might make the atmosphere less conducive to the growth of yeast. Tampons and pads that have fragrances should also be avoided because they might irritate the vaginal tissue and upset the natural equilibrium.

Moreover, nutrition and diet may be important in treating yeast infections. Maintaining a nutritious, well-balanced diet is crucial for boosting immune system performance overall. Consuming a range of fruits, vegetables, whole grains, lean meats, and healthy fats is part of this. Foods high in probiotics, such yoghurt and fermented veggies, can also be advantageous since they encourage the development of good bacteria in the vagina and gut.

Incorporating natural remedies into one's self-care routine may also be beneficial for those who experience reoccurring yeast infections and hormonal shifts. Some plants, like tea tree oil and garlic, have antibacterial qualities that can aid in the fight against yeast overgrowth. Before utilising these treatments, you should speak with a healthcare provider nevertheless, as they can have negative effects or conflict with other prescriptions.

In conclusion, especially in regard to the menstrual cycle, hormonal fluctuations can have a substantial effect on yeast infections. Variations in the amounts of progesterone and oestrogen can foster an environment that is more prone to yeast overgrowth, which can result in infections. But treating yeast infections in the setting of hormonal fluctuations necessitates a multifaceted strategy that emphasises immune system support, natural remedy incorporation, and proper vaginal hygiene. People can effectively control yeast infections and enhance general vaginal health by attending to these features.

# Hormonal Balance and Yeast Infection Management

I have direct experience with the effects that hormone imbalances can have on an individual's general health and well-being as a medical practitioner and health and wellness coach. Hormones are essential for controlling several body processes, such as digestion, immunity, and reproductive health. Our bodies' delicate environment can be upset and we become more vulnerable to infections, including yeast infections, when these hormones are out of balance.

I'll be sharing with you some methods in this chapter for managing and preventing yeast infections by preserving hormonal balance. These tactics include food adjustments, hormone therapy considerations, and lifestyle improvements. You may manage the health of your hormones and lower your risk of yeast infections by adopting these techniques into your everyday routine.

Lifestyle Modifications:

Stress, sleep deprivation, and bad habits are common in our modern lives, and they can all upset our hormonal balance. In order to preserve hormonal balance, it's critical to adopt deliberate lifestyle changes that support general health. Here are some significant lifestyle adjustments you can make:

1. Prioritize Sleep: Getting enough sleep is crucial for hormone balance. For your body to get the rest it needs to rebalance its hormones, try to get between seven and nine hours of sleep per night.

2. Manage Stress: Our hormones can be severely disrupted by ongoing stress. Include stress-reduction strategies into your everyday routine, such as deep breathing exercises, meditation, or fun hobbies.

3. Exercise Regularly: Exercise lowers inflammation in the body and aids with hormone regulation. Try to get in at least 30 minutes of

moderate-to-intense exercise most days of the week to help maintain hormonal equilibrium.

4. Practice Mindful Eating: Eating mindfully entails being aware of the cues your body gives you about hunger and fullness. Eat complete, nutrient-dense foods to fuel your body; stay away from processed foods that are loaded with artificial additives and sugar.

Dietary Changes:

Our hormonal health is directly impacted by the things we eat. Changing one's diet consciously can help maintain hormonal balance and lower the incidence of yeast infections. The following food factors should be kept in mind:

1. Avoid Foods that Promote Yeast Growth: There are some meals that can encourage the body's yeast overgrowth. These consist of processed foods, sugar-filled foods, and refined carbs. Reduce the amount of these items you eat to avoid getting yeast infections.

2. Increase Probiotic-Rich Foods: Hormonal homeostasis depends on a healthy balance of bacteria in the gut, which is maintained by probiotics. Consume foods high in probiotics, such as kimchi, kefir, yoghurt, and sauerkraut.

3. Consume Hormone-Balancing Foods: Certain meals can help control hormone levels and have the ability to balance hormones. Flaxseeds, fatty salmon, and cruciferous vegetables like broccoli and cauliflower are a few examples.

4. Stay Hydrated: Hormone balance is just one aspect of general health that is greatly impacted by drinking enough water each day. Make sure you drink eight glasses of water a day to help your hormones work at their best.

Hormone Therapy Considerations:

Hormonal abnormalities can sometimes necessitate medical attention. In addition to helping to control hormone fluctuations, hormone therapy can lower the incidence of yeast infections. Consider the following choices for hormone therapy:

1. Bioidentical Hormone Replacement Therapy (BHRT): Hormones that are structurally comparable to those the body naturally produces are used in BHRT. This treatment can assist in reestablishing hormonal equilibrium and reducing symptoms brought on by imbalances.

2. Hormonal Birth Control: Hormonal birth control may be a useful treatment for those with menstrual cycle-related hormonal abnormalities. It can lessen the risk of yeast infections and aid with hormone regulation.

3. Thyroid Hormone Replacement: Hormonal imbalances may be exacerbated by hypothyroidism, a disorder marked by an underactive thyroid. Your doctor could advise thyroid hormone replacement if your thyroid is underactive in order to bring your hormone levels back into balance.

It is crucial to remember that hormone therapy needs to be used carefully and under a doctor's supervision. They will evaluate your particular circumstances and provide a customised treatment plan that meets your requirements.

Yeast infections can be greatly decreased by putting these hormonal balance measures into practise. Recall that prevention is essential, and managing your health holistically can significantly improve your general wellbeing. Adopt these lifestyle changes, include items that balance your hormones in your diet, and, if needed, explore hormone therapy. When combined, these methods will enable you to take charge of your hormonal well-being and treat your yeast infection over the long term.

We shall go further into the relationship between yeast infections and gut health in the upcoming chapter. Watch this space to learn how to stop yeast overgrowth and preserve a healthy gut flora.

# Natural Remedies for Hormonal Balance

It's critical to address the underlying causes of any disturbances to the delicate balance between hormone production and regulation when it comes to hormonal balance. Mood swings, weight gain, exhaustion, irregular menstrual cycles, and, in certain situations, yeast infections are just a few of the symptoms that hormonal imbalances might present with. People can maintain the health of their hormones and lessen the likelihood of getting or worsening a yeast infection by using natural therapies.

For ages, traditional medical systems have utilised herbs to support hormone balance and general health. The chasteberry, or Vitex agnus-castus, is one such herb. Research indicates that this herb can increase progesterone production, which is crucial for preserving reproductive health. Chasteberry can help balance the estrogen-progesterone ratio by controlling progesterone levels. This helps relieve symptoms of hormonal imbalance and possibly lower the incidence of yeast infections.

Black cohosh is another herb that helps maintain hormonal balance. Native to North America, black cohosh has long been used to treat menopausal symptoms like mood swings and hot flashes. Since vaginal yeast overgrowth can be attributed to oestrogen abnormalities, black cohosh may help lessen the frequency and severity of yeast infections by adjusting oestrogen levels.

In addition to promoting a healthy food and way of life, supplements can help maintain hormonal balance. It has been demonstrated that omega-3 fatty acids, which are frequently included in fish oil supplements, provide a number of health advantages, including the ability to lower inflammation and maintain hormonal balance. You can lower your risk of yeast infections and promote healthy hormone synthesis by include omega-3 fatty acids in your diet.

Another important nutrient that is critical to hormone control is vitamin D. Studies have revealed a link between vitamin D insufficiency and a number of hormonal disorders, such as polycystic ovarian syndrome (PCOS). People can maintain hormonal balance and lower their risk of yeast infections by making sure they are getting enough vitamin D through supplements or sensible sun exposure.

Lifestyle behaviours are essential for supporting hormonal balance and managing yeast infections, in addition to herbs and vitamins. For instance, regular exercise can have a significant effect on the synthesis and control of hormones. Engaging in physical activity can assist to improve general well-being by lowering inflammation and stress levels. Furthermore, since obesity is linked to hormone imbalances, exercise helps with weight management, which is crucial for hormone balancing.

Maintaining hormonal health also requires effective stress management. The HPA axis, which is the delicate equilibrium between the pituitary, adrenal, and hypothalamus, can be upset by long-term stress. The synthesis and control of hormones can be impacted by disruptions to this axis, which may result in imbalances and raise the risk of yeast infections. Including stress-reduction methods like deep breathing exercises, mindfulness meditation, and soothing hobbies can help maintain hormonal balance and lower the risk of yeast infections.

Sleep is one element of hormone homeostasis that is frequently disregarded. The body's natural rhythm can be upset by getting too little or poor quality sleep, which can result in abnormalities in hormone production. Sleep has a big impact on hormones like growth hormone, melatonin, and cortisol. People can help the body's natural hormone balancing and lower their risk of yeast infections by making adequate sleep a priority.

Finally, treating any underlying mental and emotional issues is crucial in preventing hormone imbalances and yeast infections. Hormone health may suffer from unresolved trauma, long-term stress, and bad thought habits. Including self-help methods like journaling or gratitude exercises with counselling or therapy can help with stress management, enhance mental health, and maintain hormonal balance.

Managing yeast infections and achieving hormonal balance can be significantly improved by including natural therapies into your lifestyle. But it's important to keep in mind that each person is different, so what suits one person could not suit another. Speaking with a medical expert, such as a functional medicine practitioner or naturopathic doctor, may offer individualised advice and guarantee that natural remedies are properly and successfully incorporated into your daily healthcare regimen.

People can enhance their overall health and take control of their well-being by managing their yeast infections and hormones holistically. We can give our bodies the support they require to operate at their best and preserve hormonal balance by combining herbs, vitamins, and lifestyle choices.

# Hormonal Health and Self-Care Practices

I have devoted my professional life to assisting others in achieving their highest level of wellbeing as a medical doctor and health and wellness coach. Hormonal health is one area that should be prioritised but is frequently disregarded despite having a big impact on general health. The body uses hormones as chemical messengers to control a number of processes, such as mood, metabolism, and reproduction. Yeast infections are among the many health problems that can result from hormone imbalances. I will go into the significance of self-care routines for preserving hormonal balance and treating yeast infections in this chapter. You can take charge of your hormonal health and lead a fulfilling life by putting self-care and wellbeing first.

The Importance of Hormonal Health

Understanding the importance of hormonal health is essential before delving into the realm of self-care techniques. Our bodies rely heavily on hormones to control everything from our appetite to our sleep cycles. Our bodies work at their best and we feel good all around when our hormones are in balance. On the other hand, an imbalance in hormones can cause a wide range of symptoms, such as weight gain, mood fluctuations, weariness, and even yeast infections.

A form of fungus called Candida overgrows naturally in human systems and is the source of yeast infections. An environment that is favourable to Candida growth might arise when our hormonal balance is disturbed. The delicate balance of bacteria and fungus in our systems can be upset by hormonal imbalances, such as high levels of oestrogen or progesterone, which can cause an overgrowth of Candida and the consequent development of yeast infections.

Understanding Self-Care

The phrase "self-care" has become more well-known in recent years, and for good reason. It is crucial to put self-care first in our hectic, high-stress lives in order to preserve general health and wellbeing. The intentional steps we take to maintain our mental, emotional, and physical well-being are referred to as self-care. It can include a variety of pursuits, such as regular exercise, mindfulness training, and making sure we feed our bodies wholesome foods.

Importance of Self-Care in Hormonal Health

In terms of hormonal wellness, self-nurturing is crucial. We can help our body's ability to produce and maintain balanced hormone levels by practising self-care on a regular basis. The following are some significant ways that self-care routines can support hormonal balance and aid in the treatment of yeast infections:

1. Stress Reduction: Prolonged stress can have a negative impact on our hormone balance in addition to our mental health. Our bodies release the hormone cortisol during times of stress, which can upset the delicate hormonal balance of other bodily functions. Reducing cortisol levels and restoring hormonal balance can be accomplished by using stress-reduction strategies including deep breathing, meditation, or regular exercise.

2. Sleep Hygiene: Enough sleep is necessary for hormonal balance. Hormone modulation is one of the many restorative processes that our bodies go through while we sleep. We may help our bodies maintain hormonal balance by giving priority to sleep hygiene activities including making a comfortable sleep environment, adopting a soothing bedtime routine, and scheduling consistent sleep times.

3. Balanced Nutrition: Hormonal health is significantly influenced by the food we eat. Lean proteins, fruits, vegetables, healthy fats, and other whole foods can all contribute to a diet high in these nutrients, which are needed for hormone regulation and synthesis. Furthermore, some meals can help maintain a healthy balance of bacteria in our

systems, lowering the incidence of yeast infections. Examples of these foods are fermented foods like yoghurt and sauerkraut.

4. Physical Activity: Frequent exercise is good for hormone balance in addition to cardiovascular health and keeping a healthy weight. Exercise lowers stress, encourages the release of endorphins, or the feel-good chemicals, and controls insulin levels. Exercises like weight training, yoga, and walking help improve hormonal balance and lower the incidence of yeast infections.

5. Mindfulness Practices: Our hormonal health can be significantly impacted by incorporating mindfulness activities into our everyday routine. Stress can be decreased, self-awareness can be raised, and a sense of peace and balance can be encouraged by practises like journaling, deep breathing exercises, and meditation. We can assist our body's capacity to control hormone levels and treat yeast infections by calming the mind and engaging in mindfulness practises.

Prioritizing Self-Care

The next step is to make self-care a priority in our everyday life now that we know how important self-care habits are for treating yeast infections and preserving hormonal balance. Taking care of oneself is not selfish; rather, it is crucial for our wellbeing, even though it might be difficult to find the time in our hectic schedules for it.

Here are a few strategies for prioritizing self-care:

1. Set Boundaries: Saying no to obligations or activities that conflict with your wellbeing is a skill you should acquire. Give top priority to pursuits that feed your body, mind, and spirit.

2. Create a Routine: You may make sure that self-care activities are incorporated into your day by creating a regular routine. Allocate specific time for practises like mindfulness, physical activity, or unwinding with a soothing bath.

3. Seek Support: Be in the company of individuals who value and encourage your attempts at self-care. To receive a customised self-care strategy, think about consulting with a health and wellness specialist.

4. Practice Gratitude: Develop an attitude of thankfulness by recognising and enjoying life's little pleasures. Having gratitude in your life can help you think differently and feel better overall.

Conclusion

In summary, self-care routines are essential for preserving hormonal balance and controlling yeast infections. We may assist our body in producing and sustaining balanced hormone levels by making self-care a priority and taking care of our overall wellbeing. By implementing stress management techniques, getting enough sleep, maintaining a healthy diet, engaging in regular exercise, and practising mindfulness, we may make our environment less conducive to Candida overgrowth and lower our chance of developing yeast infections.

Make self-care a priority in your life and take the time to invest in yourself. By doing this, you raise your general well-being and increase the health of your hormones. Recall that taking care of oneself is essential to living a fulfilling life, not a luxury.

# Chapter 17: Yeast Infections and Gut Health

# Gut Microbiota and Yeast Infections

In order to comprehend the function of gut microbiota in managing yeast infections, one must first be able to define microbiota. The complex collection of bacteria, fungi, viruses, and other microorganisms that live in the digestive system is referred to as the gut microbiota. The health and proper operation of the digestive tract and the body as a whole are greatly dependent upon these microbes.

In a balanced state, the gut microbiota serves as a natural barrier against pathogenic organisms, such as yeast. By generating antimicrobial compounds and engaging in resource competition, the good bacteria in the gut, such as lactobacilli and bifidobacteria, aid in the regulation of yeast populations. Furthermore, maintaining the integrity of the intestinal lining is aided by a healthy gut microbiota, which stops yeast and other pathogens from entering the circulation.

Nevertheless, a number of variables may throw off the delicate balance of the gut microbiota, which could result in an overabundance of yeast and ensuing infections. Examples of well-known offenders that can eradicate both good and dangerous microorganisms and allow yeast to proliferate are antibiotics. A bad diet high in processed foods and refined sweets, long-term stress, hormone imbalances, and a compromised immune system are additional factors that can lead to gut dysbiosis and yeast overgrowth.

The immune system is a major mechanism via which gut health affects yeast infections. A large subset of the body's immune cells, referred to as gut-associated lymphoid tissue, reside in the gut (GALT). Antagonism between the gut microbiota and inflammation can make it more difficult for the immune system to fight off infections. Yeast proliferation and infections could be made possible by this compromised immune response.

Therefore, it is essential to maintain and repair a healthy gut microbiota in order to effectively control yeast infections. A mix of dietary adjustments, lifestyle alterations, and tailored supplementation can help achieve this. In order to meet each patient's specific needs and circumstances, I frequently collaborate with them to develop a personalised strategy.

Optimizing diet is the first step towards regulating gut health. The nutrients required to promote a healthy gut microbiota can be obtained through a diet high in whole, unprocessed foods, such as an abundance of fruits and vegetables, lean meats, and healthy fats. Reducing consumption of processed foods, sugar, and refined carbs is also crucial because these can feed yeast and encourage its proliferation. Additionally, I advise using fermented foods in the diet, such as kefir, sauerkraut, and yoghurt, since they contain good bacteria that can aid in the restoration of the gut microbiota.

Lifestyle adjustments can be just as important in regaining gut health as food adjustments. For example, gut dysbiosis and heightened susceptibility to infections have been associated with chronic stress. Consequently, promoting gut health and lowering the risk of yeast overgrowth can be achieved by putting stress management measures into practise, such as regular exercise, mindfulness training, and getting enough sleep.

Furthermore useful in the treatment of yeast infections and gut health issues is supplementation. One type of beneficial bacteria that can aid in reestablishing the gut microbiota is probiotics. The effects of different probiotic strains on yeast overgrowth may differ, therefore it's critical to choose a probiotic that specifically targets the type of yeast that is causing the infection. Other substances that have been demonstrated to have antifungal qualities that may help treat yeast infections include garlic, caprylic acid, and oregano oil.

In conclusion, controlling yeast infections is greatly influenced by the state of the gut microbiota. One can lessen the likelihood of yeast overgrowth and recurrence by establishing and preserving a balanced gut flora. A few effective methods for promoting gut health and avoiding yeast infections include dietary adjustments, targeted supplements, and lifestyle adjustments. As a physician and health and wellness coach, I emphasise the significance of gut health as a fundamental component of an all-encompassing and holistic strategy for managing yeast infections. People can get lasting relief from yeast infections and enjoy improved general health by maintaining a healthy gut microbiome.

# Diet and Gut Health

I have direct experience with the effects that food can have on our general health and wellbeing as a medical doctor and health and wellness coach. The relationship between nutrition and gut health is one of the main topics we address with individuals I treat for yeast infections in my clinic.

Often called the "second brain," the gut is vital to our general well-being. Trillions of bacteria, both beneficial and harmful, live there and cooperate to keep our bodies in a state of harmony and balance. Yeast infections are among the numerous health problems that can arise from a disturbance in this delicate balance.

Many people are ignorant of the impact that food decisions might have on their intestinal health. Foods have the power to either balance out the good bacteria in our stomachs or to upset the delicate balance and encourage the growth of bad bacteria, like Candida.

I will go into the significant impact that dietary decisions have on gut health and how these decisions can affect the development and treatment of yeast infections in order to provide readers a better understanding of this connection. Readers will obtain insightful knowledge from this investigation that will enable them to make knowledgeable dietary decisions, ultimately assisting in the management and prevention of yeast infections.

Understanding the Connection

Our gut health has suffered greatly as a result of the processed foods, refined sugars, and artificial additives that make up our modern diet. These food choices reduce the amount of good bacteria in our stomachs while simultaneously creating the ideal environment for dangerous germs to flourish. Our immune systems weaken as a result, leaving us more vulnerable to yeast infections.

Understanding the foods that lead to a sick gut is the first step towards using nutrition to enhance gut health. Processed foods should be consumed in moderation or never at all since they are heavy in bad fats and refined carbohydrates. These meals not only throw off the delicate bacterial balance in our stomachs, but they also give Candida the fuel it needs to grow.

Rather, I advise my patients to concentrate on including things that are good for their guts in their diet. They consist of whole grains, lean meats, fresh produce, healthy fats, and lean proteins. These foods provide a healthy gut flora since they are high in antioxidants and vital minerals.

Meal Planning for Gut Health

To ensure that we eat the correct foods to maintain gut health and effectively control yeast infections, meal planning is essential. The secret is to provide our bodies the nourishment they require and to stay away from things that encourage the growth of Candida.

A varied selection of foods from several dietary groups should be included in a balanced meal. Start by arranging colourful fruits and vegetables to fill half of your plate. Because of their high fibre content, these plant-based meals support intestinal regularity and nourish good microorganisms.

Next, concentrate on filling your plate with lean foods like beans, fish, or chicken. Protein is necessary for maintaining general health and repairing muscles. To ensure that your diet is balanced, pay attention to the portions you eat.

Incorporate whole grains into your meal planning as well, such as quinoa, brown rice, and oats. These complex carbs support intestinal health and offer long-lasting energy. Refined carbohydrates can cause blood sugar spikes and Candida overgrowth, so stay away from foods like white bread and spaghetti.

Finally, remember the importance of good fats. Nuts, avocados, and olive oil are among the foods high in omega-3 fatty acids, which are good for the gut. Additionally, these fats help to lower inflammation, which is advantageous for the treatment of yeast infections.

It's crucial to remember that there are other elements affecting our gut health besides the meals we decide to eat. Our food preparation practises can also make a big difference. Foods can be cooked to keep their nutritional content by using techniques like baking, sautéing, or steaming instead than deep-frying.

It's critical to keep an eye out for any food triggers that can make yeast infections worse when preparing meals. Although these triggers can differ from person to person, processed meals, alcohol, refined carbohydrates, and some foods containing yeast are frequently mentioned.

In summary, there is no denying the link between intestinal health and food. Readers will learn important strategies for controlling and avoiding yeast infections by investigating foods that are good for the gut and learning how dietary decisions might affect the development of these illnesses.

My mission as a physician and health and wellness coach is to enable people to take responsibility for their health and make educated decisions about their food and way of life. Our bodies may be nourished and a healthy microbiome encouraged by a gut-friendly diet that will help us heal from yeast infections and reach our best health.

# Probiotics and Gut Health

Trillions of bacteria that live in our digestive tracts make up our gut microbiome, which is vital to our general health. These microorganisms, which include viruses, bacteria, and fungus, interact with human bodies and one another to affect many bodily functions, such as immune system function and digestion. A disturbance in the delicate equilibrium of our gut microbiota can result in a number of health issues, including infections with yeast.

The fungus Candida overgrows and causes yeast infections, sometimes referred to as candidiasis. Although our bodies naturally contain Candida, an overgrowth can cause uncomfortable symptoms including burning, itching, and discharge. Antifungal drugs are frequently used in the conventional treatment of yeast infections; however, these drugs only treat the symptoms and not the underlying cause of the overgrowth.

Probiotics can help in this situation. Live bacteria and yeasts are known as probiotics, and they are good for human health in general and gut health in particular. These beneficial bacteria support healthy digestion and immune system performance by restoring and preserving the equilibrium of our gut microbiota. Probiotics are beneficial for managing yeast infections in a number of ways.

First off, by preventing the overgrowth of Candida, probiotics can aid in the prevention of yeast infections. Probiotic strains that produce lactic acid and hydrogen peroxide, such Lactobacillus acidophilus and Bifidobacterium, provide an acidic environment in the gut that inhibits the growth of Candida. Probiotics help stop Candida from growing and causing infections by encouraging this acidic environment.

Probiotics can also aid in reducing the symptoms associated with yeast infections. Certain probiotic strains can aid in reestablishing the proper balance of microorganisms in the gut, which helps lower inflammation and restore healthy vaginal flora. For those with yeast infections, this can provide much-needed comfort by reducing symptoms including burning, itching, and discharge.

It's crucial to take dosage recommendations and strain recommendations into account when selecting the best probiotics for treating yeast infections. The effects of various probiotic strains on yeast infections and gut health differ. For instance, it is well known that Lactobacillus acidophilus and Lactobacillus rhamnosus are especially good at preventing the growth of Candida. Conversely, it has been demonstrated that the beneficial yeast Saccharomyces boulardii can help heal the gut microbiota and lessen the symptoms associated with yeast infections.

It is normally advised to take probiotics on a daily basis in terms of dosage. Depending on the patient and the severity of the yeast infection, there may be differences in the ideal dosage. It is best to begin with a lesser dosage and increase it gradually if necessary. Finding the right dosage for your circumstances can be aided by speaking with a trained probiotics specialist or medical practitioner.

Probiotics can be very helpful for managing yeast infections and gut health, but it's vital to be aware that they may also interact with other drugs or medical conditions. To achieve the optimum effects, it's crucial to spread out the intake of antibiotics and probiotics because, for instance, some antibiotics can decrease the efficacy of probiotics. Furthermore, people with compromised immune systems, including those receiving chemotherapy or living with HIV, should be cautious when taking probiotics because there is a chance of infection.

To sum up, probiotics provide a safe, all-natural way to support gut health and treat yeast infections. Probiotics have the ability to reduce symptoms and prevent yeast overgrowth by balancing and repairing the gut microbiome. It's crucial to select the proper strains and adhere to dosing guidelines, though. Speak with a healthcare expert to guarantee the best outcomes and reduce any possible conflicts. Probiotics can provide long-term relief from yeast infections and enhance general wellness when included in a complete strategy to infection control.

Now that we know this, we have another effective weapon in our toolbox to combat yeast infections. We can support our body's natural defences and maintain a healthy balance in our gut microbiome by being aware of the benefits of probiotics for gut health and managing yeast infections. I urge you to learn more about probiotics and the amazing effects they may have on your overall health and wellbeing. Let's work together to eliminate yeast infections and restore intestinal health.

# Healing the Gut for Yeast Infection Management

My primary goal as a physician and health and wellness coach is to advance holistic medical treatment and wellness. I really think that treating the gut, which is the source of the illness, is the first step towards managing yeast infections. I'll discuss methods for mending the gut and enhancing gut health in this chapter to help with the treatment of yeast infections. Through the use of herbal medicines, gut-healing procedures, and lifestyle changes, readers will be given invaluable tools to take back control of their health.

The stomach, sometimes called the second brain, is essential to our general health. In addition to digesting and absorbing nutrients, the gut microbiota is home to trillions of microorganisms. These microbes have a significant effect on our digestion, mental health, immune system, and even skin. Many health problems, including yeast infections, can result from a disruption in this microbiota's balance.

Making changes to one's lifestyle is one of the first stages toward intestinal healing. This include eating a nutritious, well-balanced diet, managing your stress, and exercising frequently. A diet high in whole foods, like fruits, vegetables, lean meats, and healthy fats, can supply vital nutrients and support a gut environment that is conducive to health. Alcohol, refined carbohydrates, and processed meals should all be consumed in moderation as these might encourage the growth of dangerous germs and yeast.

Furthermore, gut health is directly impacted by stress. Prolonged stress can throw the body's microbiota out of balance and make inflammation worse. Including stress-relieving activities in your everyday routine is essential. This can involve practising yoga, deep breathing techniques, meditation, or relaxing pastimes.

In addition, frequent exercise helps to maintain a healthy stomach by strengthening the immune system and lowering inflammation. Most days of the week, try to get in at least 30 minutes of moderate-intensity activity, like brisk walking or cycling.

Herbal therapies, in addition to lifestyle improvements, can be quite effective in promoting gut healing. Strong antibacterial and anti-inflammatory qualities found in certain herbs can aid in reestablishing the equilibrium of the gut microbiota. For example, ginger and turmeric have strong anti-inflammatory properties, and oregano oil and grapefruit seed extract can function as natural antifungals.

To find out the right amount and length of time to use these herbs, speak with a healthcare provider or herbalist. In order to support general gut health, they can also help you choose other advantageous herbs and supplements, like digestive enzymes and probiotics.

Moreover, healing can be accelerated by adhering to a gut-healing routine. Usually, this strategy calls for a temporary elimination of substances that cause inflammation and damage to the gut, including dairy, gluten, and processed meals. This permits the intestines to mend and renew. To evaluate their impact on gut health and tolerance, these foods can be progressively reintroduced after the exclusion phase.

It is crucial to concentrate on feeding the gut with nutrient-dense foods during this therapy. For instance, bone broth has high levels of collagen and amino acids that aid in the regeneration of the gut lining. Fermented foods, including kefir and sauerkraut, contain good bacteria that can aid in microbiota rebalancing.

Furthermore, supplementing with gut-healing foods like aloe vera and L-glutamine might help the gut lining mend even more. These supplements function as calming and shielding substances, lowering inflammation and encouraging the development of wholesome intestinal cells.

It is important to stress that mending the gut requires commitment and time. It is a long-term commitment to holistic wellness rather than a fast remedy. Finding the ideal ratio of dietary changes, herbal therapies, and gut-healing procedures may take some trial and error for each person.

To sum up, treating yeast infections requires first tending to the gut. People can help restore a healthy gut microbiota and enhance their general well-being by adopting lifestyle changes, using herbal medicines, and adhering to gut-healing procedures. Recall that every person's path to ideal gut health is different, but that long-term health and the ability to treat yeast infections are both achievable with persistence and patience.

# Chapter 18: Yeast Infections and Allergies

# Allergies and Yeast Infections: Understanding the Connection

We will go into more depth about this relationship in this subchapter, including how allergies may exacerbate yeast overgrowth and how symptoms may coexist. By doing this, we seek to clarify the intricacies of yeast infections and give you a thorough grasp of the potential role allergies may play in their emergence.

Let's start by defining allergies and discussing how the body reacts to them. An allergic reaction is an overreaction by the immune system to normally harmless things like dust mites, pollen, or specific foods. Upon encountering these triggers, an individual with allergies experiences a reaction from their immune system, which releases a series of chemicals and hormones to protect against the perceived threat.

The generation of Immunoglobulin E (IgE), a class of antibody that attaches to allergens and releases histamine, is a part of the immunological response to allergies. The traditional allergy symptoms, such sneezing, itching, and swelling, are brought on by histamine. The body is trying to get rid of the perceived threat and get back to balance by exhibiting these symptoms.

Let's now explore the relationship between yeast infections and allergies. The fact that a complex ecosystem of potentially hazardous as well as helpful microbes resides within our bodies is an important fact to grasp. Yeast, fungus, viruses, and bacteria are some of these microbes. These species coexist peacefully in the regular course of things, preserving a delicate balance that is vital to our health and welfare.

But a few things have the potential to upset this equilibrium, which would then cause yeast—especially Candida species—to overproliferate. A form of fungus called Candida is present in our bodies naturally and is mainly found in the mouth, throat, genital area, and digestive tract. A yeast infection can result from the proliferation of Candida when the balance is upset.

An immune system that is compromised is one of the main causes of yeast development. This is where the significance of the connection to allergies arises. The immune system can eventually become overburdened and compromised if it is continuously mounting an excessive defence against allergens. Due to the immune system's compromised state, Candida is able to proliferate and spread, leading to an infection.

Furthermore, an environment that is favourable to yeast overgrowth can be created within the body by the immunological response that allergies elicit. It has been demonstrated that histamine, the primary cause of allergy symptoms, increases the gut lining's permeability. Leaky gut syndrome, which is characterised by increased permeability, can let dangerous substances like Candida enter the bloodstream and disrupt multiple bodily systems.

It's interesting to note that studies have linked allergies to the existence of Candida species. According to a research in the Journal of Medical Microbiology, nasal passage Candida colonisation is more common in people with allergies, especially in those who have asthma and allergic rhinitis. This colonisation may act as a reservoir for Candida, which could aggravate allergy symptoms and lead to recurring infections.

Moreover, it may be more difficult to diagnose and treat yeast infections and allergies because of their similar symptoms. Symptoms like itching, redness, and inflammation are prevalent in people with yeast infections and are also classic indicators of an allergic reaction. This overlap may result in an incorrect diagnosis or a delay in receiving the proper care, exacerbating the patient's pain and aggravation.

These results highlight the importance of treating yeast infections and allergies in their whole when treating these illnesses. We can lessen the strain on the immune system and strengthen the body's defences against yeast overgrowth by managing allergies well. This could entail recognising and avoiding allergens, changing one's lifestyle to limit exposure, and utilising the right medical treatments to relieve symptoms.

Furthermore, it's critical to treat yeast infections while taking allergies into account as a possible contributing factor. By treating underlying allergens, we can improve treatment efficacy and lower the chance of recurrence by altering the body's environment to one that is less supportive of yeast development.

In summary, there is a complicated and nuanced relationship between allergies and yeast infections. In order to effectively manage yeast overgrowth and allergies, it is important to recognise how these illnesses might overlap in symptoms. We can provide people a guide for managing yeast infections completely and give them the tools they need to take back control of their health and wellbeing by adopting a comprehensive approach that addresses both allergies and yeast infections.

# Identifying and Managing Allergies

Let's start by taking a closer look at common allergens that may trigger yeast infections. These allergens can vary from person to person, but there are a few that tend to affect a larger portion of the population. The most prevalent allergens associated with yeast infections include:

1. Food Allergies: Food allergies are common in people who simultaneously have yeast infections. Dairy, sugar, maize, gluten, and soy are common offenders. These meals may encourage the body's yeast growth, which could worsen inflammation and pain.

2. Environmental Allergens: A number of environmental allergens, including mould, dust mites, pet dander, and pollen, can exacerbate yeast infections. In those who are vulnerable, these allergens may set off an immunological reaction that results in inflammation and a higher risk of infection.

3. Chemical Sensitivities: Yeast infections can be made worse by a number of substances that are included in common products including cleaning supplies, personal care items, and even some drugs. Certain people have been documented to experience hypersensitive reactions to fragrances, colours, and preservatives, which increases their vulnerability to yeast overgrowth.

The first step in managing these allergies effectively is identifying them. Thankfully, there are a number of allergy testing techniques that can assist in identifying allergens that might be causing your yeast infections. Here are some of the most popular techniques for testing:

1. Skin Prick Test: Among the most popular allergy tests is this one. Various allergens are applied topically in little doses, usually to the back or forearm. There will be a tiny welt or hive there if you are allergic to any of the ingredients. This test is comparatively non-invasive and can yield results right away.

2. Blood Test: A blood test is another reliable way to test for allergies since it counts the quantity of particular antibodies in your

blood. This makes it easier to determine whether specific allergens are causing your body to mount an immunological response. Although blood tests can be more costly and take longer to get findings, they are helpful in the diagnosis of allergies that are difficult to identify with other techniques.

3. Elimination Diet: An elimination diet can be very instructive for people who are suspected of having food allergies. This is temporarily cutting out items like gluten, dairy, and soy from your diet that are known to be common allergies. You can determine whether there is a connection between eating a specific food and the recurrence of your yeast infection symptoms by cautiously reintroducing these foods one at a time.

Making lifestyle changes to control your allergies and lower your chance of developing yeast infections is the next step after determining which allergens trigger you. The following tactics may be useful:

1. Avoiding Allergens: Preventing exposure to the allergens you have identified is the best method to prevent allergic responses. Changing your diet, using hypoallergenic cleaning and personal care products, and taking precautions to reduce your exposure to environmental allergens—like using air purifiers or keeping windows closed during pollen season—may all be part of this.

2. Boosting Immune Function: Proper immune system function is necessary to control allergies and avoid yeast infections. Put your attention on strengthening your immune system with a healthy diet, consistent exercise, stress reduction methods, and enough sleep.

3. Probiotics and Prebiotics: You can lower your risk of yeast overgrowth and help balance your body's natural flora by increasing the beneficial bacteria in your stomach. Include items high in probiotics in your diet, such as fermented vegetables and yoghurt. Foods high in prebiotics, including onions and garlic, can help encourage the growth of good bacteria.

4. Stress Management: Prolonged stress can impair immunity and raise the possibility of infections and allergic responses. Include stress-reduction strategies in your everyday routine, such as deep breathing exercises, meditation, and relaxing pursuits of pleasure.

5. Self-Care Practices: Taking good care of your mental and physical health is crucial to controlling your allergies and avoiding yeast infections. Make self-care routines a priority, including getting enough sleep, maintaining good hygiene, exercising frequently, and asking for help from friends, family, or a therapist when necessary.

You are controlling your yeast infections proactively by recognising and treating your sensitivities. You can greatly lessen the frequency and intensity of your symptoms while enhancing your general health and fitness by changing your way of living. Recall that holistic medicine aims to restore a state of harmonious balance in your body and mind by treating not just the symptoms but also their underlying causes. Remain dedicated to your path and have faith in your ability to take charge of your health again.

# Addressing Allergies and Yeast Infections Simultaneously

Let's start by discussing the meaning and background of allergies and yeast infections. Allergies, sometimes referred to as allergic reactions, happen when the body's defences misinterpret a substance that is safe and trigger an immunological response against it. Numerous symptoms, including as sneezing, itching, watery eyes, nasal congestion, and skin rashes, may appear as a result of this. Pollen, dust mites, pet dander, certain foods, and bug stings are a few frequent allergens.

Conversely, an overabundance of the fungus Candida in the vagina causes yeast infections, more especially vaginal yeast infections in this case. Though an overgrowth and subsequent infection can result from an imbalance in the vaginal ecology, candida is a naturally occurring resident of the body. Vaginal yeast infections can cause burning, itching, and unusual discharge as symptoms.

Now that we are clear on what allergies and yeast infections are, let's look at how to treat and manage both at the same time. Accurate diagnosis is the first step towards resolving this twin burden. To guarantee the right course of therapy, it's critical to differentiate between yeast infections and allergic reactions. A complete medical evaluation that includes a detailed medical history, a physical examination, and diagnostic procedures like vaginal swabs and allergy testing can be used to do this.

Treatment solutions can be customised to address yeast infections and allergies once the diagnosis has been made. Avoiding allergens is the main strategy for treating allergies. Symptoms can be considerably reduced by identifying allergies and limiting exposure to them. This could entail taking precautions like closing windows during pollen season, covering pillows and mattresses with dust mite covers, and avoiding foods that are known to cause allergies. When avoiding allergens isn't enough, doctors may prescribe antihistamines, nasal sprays, and eye drops to treat the symptoms.

Antifungal drugs are usually used in the treatment of yeast infections. Depending on the infection's location and intensity, they can be used topically, orally, or vaginally. For milder infections, over-the-counter antifungal creams and suppositories are available; for more severe instances, prescription oral drugs could be required. To guarantee total eradication of the infection, it is crucial to adhere to the recommended treatment plan and finish the entire term of medicine.

Apart from targeted therapies, lifestyle adjustments and preventive actions can aid in the management of yeast infections and allergies. First and foremost, proper hygiene is essential. This entails wearing breathable underwear composed of natural fibres, refraining from using scented products, and routinely bathing and drying the genital area. Second, keeping a nutritious, well-balanced diet is crucial. Excessive sugar intake is one dietary element that can promote the growth of Candida and raise the risk of yeast infections. Seeking advice from a dietician or nutritionist can be quite beneficial in this context.

Moreover, treating allergies and yeast infections can both benefit from the use of stress management strategies. Immune system dysregulation has been connected to stress, which can make both illnesses worse. Deep breathing exercises, yoga, and mindfulness meditation are a few practises that might help reduce stress and improve general wellbeing. A strong immune system is also greatly aided by getting enough sleep, exercising frequently, and drinking the right amount of water.

As a holistic medical professional, I think treating the underlying causes of illnesses is more important than just treating their symptoms. Investigating underlying variables that can contribute to the prevalence of allergies and yeast infections is crucial. Hormonal abnormalities, compromised immunity, dysbiosis in the gastrointestinal tract, and persistent inflammation are a few of them. You can manage allergies and yeast infections and eventually lessen their frequency and severity by treating these underlying causes with dietary adjustments, targeted supplementation, and lifestyle changes.

In conclusion, treating yeast infections and allergies at the same time necessitates a thorough and diversified strategy. The management of these illnesses has been covered in this subchapter, along with treatment choices, preventative measures, and lifestyle changes that can improve general health and wellbeing. People can alleviate symptoms and enhance their quality of life by comprehending the intricate relationship between yeast infections and allergies and managing them holistically. As usual, seeking individualised advice and support from a healthcare expert is crucial.

# Seeking Professional Guidance for Allergies and Yeast Infections

I have always supported a holistic approach to healthcare and wellbeing as a medical practitioner and health and wellness coach. While home remedies and self-care practises can be useful in controlling some medical illnesses, it is crucial to recognise that professional help is necessary when dealing with allergies and yeast infections. This chapter will examine the reasons that obtaining advice from experts and medical professionals is essential to thorough treatment and effective management of certain illnesses.

1. Understanding the Complexity of Allergies and Yeast Infections:
Yeast infections and allergies are complicated diseases with a wide range of underlying causes, triggers, and symptoms. Even while there are over-the-counter drugs and natural cures accessible, it's crucial to recognise that what works for one individual may not necessarily work for another. Moreover, not all signs and symptoms of yeast infections and allergies may be apparent or identifiable right away.

For example, allergies can be moderate to severe and are brought on by a variety of allergens, including food, pollen, pet dander, and medications. Likewise, an overabundance of the fungus Candida can result in yeast infections, which can impact various body regions such as the mouth, stomach, vagina, and blood vessels.

Because many illnesses are complex, consulting a professional is necessary to precisely identify the underlying cause and choose the best course of action.

2. Identifying when to Consult Healthcare Professionals:
Managing allergies and yeast infections successfully requires knowing when to seek medical advice. The following symptoms point to the need for expert advice:
a. Chronic or Recurrent Symptoms:

It is crucial to speak with a healthcare provider if you experience persistent or recurrent allergy or yeast infection symptoms. Chronic symptoms can include recurrent episodes of yeast infections, allergies-related skin rashes or itching, and persistent sneezing.

These signs could point to an underlying problem that needs to be thoroughly assessed and treated with a customised strategy. Based on your unique needs, a healthcare provider can perform a comprehensive evaluation, prescribe diagnostic tests, and create a suitable management plan.

b. Severe or Debilitating Symptoms:

Allergies and yeast infections can occasionally cause severe or incapacitating symptoms. For example, severe allergic reactions can result in anaphylaxis, which is a potentially fatal illness that needs to be treated right away. Similar to this, persistent or severe yeast infections can cause issues and call for medical attention.

Seeking immediate medical attention is crucial if you develop severe symptoms including trouble breathing, swelling of the lips or throat, excruciating pain, or unbearable discomfort. Health care providers are equipped with the knowledge and skills necessary to manage these circumstances and can offer the right measures to protect your safety and wellbeing.

c. Lack of Response to Self-Care Strategies:

For moderate allergies and yeast infections, self-care techniques such as using over-the-counter drugs and home remedies can offer temporary relief. It is imperative that you speak with a healthcare provider if, after taking these steps, your symptoms continue or get worse.

Based on your particular illness and medical history, a healthcare professional can determine whether the treatment plan needs to be modified, investigate possible underlying causes, and suggest more focused therapies. Keep in mind that each person has a different body, so what works for one person might not work for another.

3. The Role of Specialists in Allergies and Yeast Infections:

While general practitioners can diagnose and treat yeast infections and allergies, there may be situations when a specialist's knowledge is needed. Specialists can offer a more thorough approach to care and guarantee that all facets of your ailment are appropriately handled when they are involved.

a. Allergists/Immunologists:

Immunologists and allergists are experts in the identification and treatment of immune system problems and allergies. They are quite knowledgeable about the different allergens, triggers, and immunological reactions connected to allergies. Seeing an allergist or immunologist can help determine the precise causes for your allergies and create a customised treatment plan that may include immunotherapy if needed as well as allergy avoidance techniques.

b. Gynecologists/Urologists:

If someone is suffering from recurring vaginal yeast infections, it is advisable for women to see a gynaecologist and for males to see a urologist. To address the underlying reasons, these professionals can give tailored therapy options and a more focused evaluation of the issue.

c. Dermatologists:

Rashes, hives, and other skin-related symptoms are common manifestations of allergic reactions. Dermatologists are experts in the diagnosis and treatment of a wide range of skin disorders, including allergy-related ones. Seeing a dermatologist can guarantee a complete evaluation and effective treatment of your allergies if they emerge as skin symptoms.

4. The Benefits of Professional Guidance for Comprehensive Care:

When it comes to thorough treatment and management, consulting a specialist for yeast infections and allergies might offer the following advantages:

a. Accurate Diagnosis:

Accurate diagnosis of yeast infections and allergies is possible with the knowledge and experience of healthcare professionals and specialists. With thorough assessments that include physical examinations, medical histories, and any required diagnostic testing, they are able to detect any coexisting disorders that may need to be managed as well as identify the underlying causes.

b. Tailored Treatment Plans:

Healthcare providers can create individualised treatment programmes based on your unique needs and medical history once an accurate diagnosis has been made. This could involve a mix of prescription drugs, dietary adjustments, and preventative measures. A customised strategy maximises the efficacy of treatment by addressing every facet of your disease.

c. Access to Specialized Interventions:

Access to specific interventions may be provided by healthcare professionals based on the severity or complexity of your yeast infections or allergies. This can involve antifungal treatments for yeast infections or immunotherapy for allergies. These specialist treatments are intended to address the underlying causes of your ailment and offer long-term care and relief.

d. Continuous Monitoring and Follow-up:

Under the direction of a professional, you may be sure that your condition will be properly managed throughout time with ongoing monitoring. Medical specialists are able to monitor how your therapy is going, assess any changes in your symptoms, and modify your management strategy as needed. Having follow-up appointments on a regular basis guarantees that you receive continued assistance for the best possible care and gives you the chance to address any questions or concerns.

In summary, for complete care and the best possible management of yeast infections and allergies, consulting a professional is essential. These disorders can have a wide range of underlying causes and symptoms since they are complex. You can guarantee an accurate diagnosis, customised treatment plans, access to expert therapies, and ongoing monitoring to achieve long-term comfort and well-being by speaking with medical professionals and specialists. Recall that expert advice is an investment in your general health and well-being, and that your health is a valuable resource.

# Chapter 19: Yeast Infections and Autoimmune Disorders

# Autoimmune Disorders and Yeast Infections

Understanding each of the two terms on their own is essential to understanding the relationship between autoimmune diseases and yeast infections. When the immune system, which is meant to defend the body against dangerous invaders, unintentionally targets healthy cells within the body, autoimmune illnesses result. This syndrome impairs the regular operation of tissues and organs and causes persistent inflammation. Among many others, lupus, multiple sclerosis, celiac disease, and rheumatoid arthritis are among the most prevalent autoimmune diseases.

Conversely, yeast infections—more especially, Candida overgrowth—occur when the body's delicate microbe balance is upset, which permits the yeast to develop quickly. Our bodies naturally contain a type of fungus called candida, which is most common in the vaginal area, the digestive tract, and the folds of our skin. Normally, Candida is kept at bay by the immune system and other helpful microbes. But several things can tip the scales in favour of Candida overgrowth, including hormone abnormalities, antibiotics, weakened immune systems, and high-sugar diets.

Let's now explore the complex interaction between these two circumstances. The delicate balance of microbes, including Candida, in our bodies is critically dependent on the immune system. When it works correctly, it may recognise dangerous infections and get rid of them, controlling them. But in autoimmune diseases, the immune system goes into overdrive and attacks healthy cells as well, making the body open to a variety of infections, including an overabundance of yeast.

Studies have indicated that immune responses against Candida are frequently weakened in people with autoimmune diseases. According to a 2015 study by Dr. Shenoy et al., patients with rheumatoid arthritis had higher levels of antibodies against the fungus Candida, suggesting a dysregulated immune response. Furthermore, in comparison to healthy persons, patients with autoimmune thyroiditis—a common autoimmune disorder—exhibited greater rates of Candida colonisation in their oral cavities, according to a 2019 study published in the Journal of Microbiology and Infectious Diseases.

There are other reasons that can be linked to the underlying processes of this impaired immune response. The immune system is always activated in autoimmune illnesses, generating pro-inflammatory cytokines that spread inflammation throughout the body. This persistent inflammation makes it more difficult for the immune system to fight off infections like Candida. Furthermore, the immune system can be further weakened by several drugs used to treat autoimmune diseases, such as immunosuppressants and corticosteroids, which increases a person's susceptibility to yeast infections.

Moreover, hormonal abnormalities are a common component of autoimmune illnesses and may potentially contribute to yeast overgrowth. The body's ability to control the growth of Candida is greatly influenced by hormones. For instance, oestrogen may encourage Candida to cling to vaginal cells, raising the incidence of vaginal yeast infections in females. Hormonal imbalances are linked to a number of autoimmune diseases, including lupus and thyroid disorders, which increases the risk of developing yeast infections.

It's also critical to remember that long-term stress can weaken the immune system and throw off the delicate balance of microbes in the body. Chronic stress is common in people with autoimmune illnesses. Stress hormones like cortisol can erode immune system defences and foster an atmosphere that's ideal for Candida overgrowth.

Taking a thorough strategy is essential for handling yeast infections and autoimmune illnesses because of their intricate interactions. Conventional medical therapies usually involve the use of pharmaceuticals, such as antifungals and anti-inflammatory agents, to manage symptoms. Although these therapies might offer short-term respite, they don't deal with the fundamental causes of these illnesses.

As a holistic medical professional, I treat autoimmune diseases and yeast infections by addressing their underlying causes and fostering general wellness. This calls for a multimodal strategy that includes dietary changes, stress reduction methods, lifestyle adjustments, and natural therapies that boost the immune system and help the body regain its equilibrium.

Changes in lifestyle are crucial first and foremost. This includes practises that have been demonstrated to modify immune function and reduce inflammation, such as deep breathing exercises, yoga, and meditation, as well as stress reduction strategies. In addition, maintaining a healthy weight, getting enough sleep, and exercising frequently are essential for boosting immunity and controlling hormone levels.

Reducing sugar intake and following an anti-inflammatory diet are crucial dietary strategies. A high-sugar diet can promote the growth of Candida and impair immunological responses, according to studies. Rather, concentrate on eating entire meals, such as an abundance of fresh fruits and vegetables, lean meats, and good fats. Foods high in probiotics, like kefir, yoghurt, and fermented veggies, can also help restore the proper balance of good bacteria in the stomach, preventing the overgrowth of yeast.

Supplements may also help the body's immune system and restore equilibrium. It has been demonstrated that zinc, vitamin C, and omega-3 fatty acids have immunomodulatory and anti-inflammatory properties. Furthermore, when taken properly, several herbs, such pau d'arco, oregano, and garlic, have antifungal qualities that can help reduce yeast overgrowth.

In summary, there is a nuanced and intricate relationship between yeast infections and autoimmune diseases. In addition to impairing immune function, autoimmune diseases can provide an atmosphere that encourages the growth of yeast. Through the implementation of a comprehensive strategy that encompasses dietary adjustments, stress reduction techniques, lifestyle adjustments, and natural therapies, people can effectively manage both illnesses and reestablish bodily balance. I'm still dedicated to assisting my patients in mastering yeast infections and achieving optimal health and wellness in my capacity as a medical doctor and health and wellness coach.

# Managing Autoimmune Disorders and Yeast Infections

When the immune system unintentionally targets and destroys healthy cells in the body, autoimmune diseases result. An overreaction of the immune system can result in chronic inflammation and a number of symptoms, including weariness, discomfort in the joints, and digestive problems. On the other hand, an overabundance of Candida albicans, a form of yeast that is normally present in our bodies, causes yeast infections, sometimes referred to as candidiasis. Symptoms like burning, itching, and discharge might be signs of an excess of yeast that occurs when the delicate balance between bacteria and yeast is upset.

Many people are unaware of the close relationship that exists between yeast infections and autoimmune illnesses. Research has indicated that immunocompromised patients with autoimmune illnesses are more vulnerable to yeast infections. Moreover, the persistent inflammation linked to autoimmune diseases creates a perfect setting for yeast growth.

Let's now explore the tactics that will enable you to successfully handle both scenarios. Remember that these are only suggestions, and that before making any big changes to your lifestyle or course of treatment, you should speak with your doctor or a holistic health specialist.

Lifestyle Modifications:

Making specific lifestyle adjustments is one of the first steps towards simultaneously controlling yeast infections and autoimmune illnesses. Your immune system will be strengthened and your general health will be supported by these adjustments.

Setting stress management as a top priority is crucial. Your immune system may be negatively impacted by prolonged stress, which raises your chance of developing yeast infections and autoimmune diseases.

Deep breathing exercises, yoga, meditation, and spending time in nature are a few practises that can help reduce stress and enhance general wellbeing.

Exercise on a regular basis is also essential. In addition to strengthening the immune system, exercise also helps control hormones and enhance blood flow. On most days of the week, try to get in at least 30 minutes of moderate-intensity exercise. It can be as easy as riding a bike, swimming, or walking. To incorporate enjoyable activities into your schedule, choose ones that you look forward to.

Dietary Changes:

Nutrition is important for both autoimmune disease management and yeast overgrowth prevention. You can integrate the following food modifications into your routine:

1. Anti-inflammatory Foods: Your diet should be centred on including full, unprocessed foods such fruits, vegetables, whole grains, lean meats, and healthy fats. Antioxidants, vitamins, and minerals abound in these foods and can help lower inflammation.

2. Avoid Trigger Foods: Both yeast infections and autoimmune diseases can be brought on by or made worse by specific foods. Processed meals, refined sugars, gluten, alcohol, and dairy products are frequently identified as perpetrators. To find your unique trigger foods, try an exclusion diet or speak with a trained nutritionist.

3. Probiotics: Probiotics are good bacteria that aid in reestablishing the equilibrium of the gut flora, which is necessary for a strong immune system. Include items that have undergone fermentation in your diet, such as kefir, yoghurt, sauerkraut, or kimchi. To promote the health of your gut, you can also take a high-quality probiotic supplement.

4. Sugar Reduction: Since sugar is what Candida yeast loves, cutting back on sugar is essential to treating yeast infections. Stevia or monk fruit are good natural sweeteners; stay away from sodas, candy, processed foods, and sugary drinks.

Immune Support Techniques:

Improving your immune system is crucial for controlling yeast infections and autoimmune diseases. The following are some practical immune-boosting methods:

1. Supplements: There are substances that can help lower inflammation and boost your immune system. Zinc, vitamin C, vitamin D, and omega-3 fatty acids are some of the best nutrients for supporting the immune system. To find the ideal dosage for you, consult a holistic health specialist or your healthcare practitioner.

2. Herbal Remedies: Numerous herbs contain antifungal and immune-stimulating qualities that can help your body combat yeast infections and autoimmune diseases. Garlic, oregano oil, pau d'arco, and caprylic acid are a few common alternatives. To guarantee the correct application and dosage of these herbs, it is imperative to speak with an experienced herbalist or naturopath.

3. Sleep and Rest: Getting enough sleep is essential for your immune system to perform at its best. Every night, try to get between seven and nine hours of good sleep. Prioritize relaxing methods like stretching or meditation before bed.

In summary, a thorough and all-encompassing approach is necessary for the simultaneous management of yeast infections and autoimmune illnesses. Through the application of dietary adjustments, immune support strategies, and lifestyle modifications, you can successfully manage symptoms, lower inflammation, and enhance your general health. To create a personalised management plan, keep in mind that working with your healthcare physician or a holistic health professional is crucial. By working together, we can create a path toward total management of yeast infections and enhanced life quality.

# Coordinating Care With Healthcare Professionals

Both yeast infections and autoimmune diseases are complicated ailments that call for a multimodal approach to therapy. They frequently take on many forms and impact various bodily systems and organs. This necessitates an all-encompassing strategy that takes into account the psychological and emotional as well as the physical symptoms of the illness. Together, healthcare providers can bring their distinct expertise and viewpoints to bear on developing a treatment strategy that is customised to each patient's needs.

Addressing the root causes of yeast infections and autoimmune diseases is one of the main advantages of a multidisciplinary approach. A holistic approach seeks to determine and treat the underlying causes of these diseases, whereas conventional medicine frequently concentrates on treating their symptoms. We may explore the underlying causes of these disorders, including hormonal imbalances, gut dysbiosis, and chronic stress, in greater detail by bringing in the knowledge of experts from alternative therapies, psychology, functional medicine, and nutrition. This enables us to create specialised therapy regimens that support long-term recovery and wellness in addition to symptom relief.

In order to perform comprehensive evaluations and diagnostic testing, functional medicine practitioners and I frequently work together in my clinic. This aids in the detection of any bodily dysfunctions or imbalances that might be causing an autoimmune disease or yeast infection. This data, along with the patient's symptoms and medical history, help us create a more precise and individualised therapy plan.

Nutrition is one area where a multidisciplinary approach can be especially helpful. With autoimmune diseases and yeast infections, diet is very important because specific foods can make symptoms worse or better. Together with a nutritionist or dietician, we may create a customised meal plan that meets each patient's unique requirements. This could entail introducing foods that repair the gut, removing foods that cause inflammation, and making sure you're getting enough nutrients. We can assist the body's natural healing processes and enhance general health by treating dietary deficiencies and fostering a healthy gut microbiota.

A thorough treatment strategy should address the psychological and emotional components of yeast infections and autoimmune illnesses in addition to the physical symptoms. These disorders can be emotionally and mentally taxing, frequently leading to feelings of anxiety, frustration, and loneliness. Patients who engage with a psychologist or counsellor can obtain the necessary assistance and guidance to effectively manage these issues. This can entail treating any underlying emotional problems that might be aggravating symptoms as well as developing coping mechanisms and stress-reduction tactics. We can assist patients in improving their general quality of life and sense of well-being by addressing the mind-body link.

Additionally, complementary therapies are beneficial in the treatment of yeast infections and autoimmune diseases. Acupuncture, massage, and herbal medicine are among the techniques that might help reduce symptoms and encourage the body's inherent healing process. Collaborating with practitioners of these modalities allows us to provide patients a more all-encompassing and integrated approach to their treatment.

For autoimmune diseases and yeast infections to be effectively managed, care coordination with medical specialists is crucial. By bringing together experts from different domains, we can access a multitude of knowledge and experience to develop a treatment plan that supports the body's own healing processes while addressing the underlying causes of these disorders. Patients can receive the customised care they require through a multidisciplinary approach, which supports long-term healing and maximum wellness.

# Empowering Self-Advocacy and Education

In order to empower oneself, one must take an active role in the healthcare process. The days of patients blindly following their doctor's orders are long gone. Patients should now feel free to clarify things, ask questions, and take an active role in making decisions. Patients may guarantee they are getting the greatest care available and regain control over their health by doing this.

I welcome questions from my patients during their sessions in my clinic. I think it's critical that people are well informed about their ailment, available treatments, and any adverse effects. Patients can make decisions that are in line with their values and personal goals by actively participating in a discourse with their healthcare professionals.

Patients can educate themselves on their problems in addition to talking with their healthcare providers. This can be accomplished in a number of ways, including reading reputable publications, going to informative workshops, and joining support groups. Patients can better manage the intricacies of their healthcare journey by developing a deeper grasp of their diseases.

For instance, a lot of people might not be aware of the risk factors, treatment alternatives, or underlying causes of yeast infections. Patients might feel more empowered and take action to effectively manage their symptoms by learning more about the disease.

I have compiled thorough and current information regarding yeast infections in this book to aid in the teaching process. Readers will get the knowledge necessary to make educated decisions regarding their own heath through a thorough examination of the causes, symptoms, and possible treatment options.

Additionally, readers will learn about the different lifestyle changes that can help stop recurrent yeast infections. The book discusses many self-care strategies that can be used in conjunction with medical therapies, such as stress management methods and dietary adjustments. Realizing the value of getting a second opinion is one of the cornerstones of empowering self-advocacy. Healthcare professionals work hard to give patients the best care possible, but it's vital to recognise that medical knowledge is always changing and that various physicians may have different opinions and methods to treatment. Patients can obtain new insights and feel more at ease knowing they have considered every possibility by getting a second opinion.

In my practise, I frequently advise patients to consult with other doctors before making important treatment decisions. I am aware that there may be several routes to wellness and that healthcare can be complicated. Patients can make well-informed decisions that are consistent with their individual tastes and values by considering many points of view.

Knowing one's own rights as a patient is a crucial component of self-advocacy. Patients have the right to request a copy of their test findings, view their medical records, and decide how they will be treated in many different nations. Patients can express their autonomy and actively engage in their healthcare journey by being aware of these rights.

I also discuss the value of psychosocial support in the treatment of yeast infections in this book. Living with a chronic illness can have a major psychological and emotional impact, which is sometimes disregarded yet is very important. Readers will be able to address the emotional components of their condition and take steps toward enhancing their general well-being by receiving tools and coping skills.

Through education and self-advocacy, readers of this book will take an active role in their own healthcare by empowering themselves. They'll learn more about the specific ailments they have, available treatments, and ways to change their way of life. Equipped with an understanding and a feeling of mastery, readers will be capable of making knowledgeable choices and proficiently handling their yeast infections.

My ultimate objective is to provide people the tools they need to take control of their health and wellbeing. People may prosper and live their best lives by getting educated, speaking out for themselves, and receiving healthcare from a holistic perspective. I have no doubt that this book will give readers the resources they require to accomplish that.

# Chapter 20: Thriving Beyond Yeast Infections

# Sustaining Progress and Preventing Recurrence

It's critical to realise that treating persistent yeast infections is a complex process that calls both ongoing commitment and a well-thought-out strategy. I'll guide you through tactics in this section that will help you maintain your progress and stop yeast infections from coming back.

Long-Term Maintenance Plans:

The creation of a long-term maintenance plan is one of the most important elements in maintaining development. This plan, which will include several components catered to your individual needs, will act as a guide for your continued management of yeast infections. Among these components could be:

1. Lifestyle Modifications: It's essential to make specific lifestyle changes to stop recurrent yeast infections. This could entail adjustments to one's diet, exercise regimen, and stress-reduction strategies. Reassessing and modifying your way of living gives your body the ability to keep a balanced state and avoid yeast overgrowth.

2. Food and Diet Planning: It's no secret that our susceptibility to yeast infections and other health issues is greatly influenced by the foods we eat. Our team of experts will provide you a customised food and diet plan as part of your long-term maintenance plan that helps avoid yeast overgrowth and fosters a gut-friendly environment. This strategy can include cutting back on sugar and processed carbs, consuming more fibre, adding foods high in probiotics, and avoiding trigger foods that might encourage yeast overgrowth.

3. Counseling and Psychology Related Techniques: I sincerely believe in the mind-body link and acknowledge the influence that psychological variables can have on our physical health as a holistic healthcare practitioner. A long-term maintenance strategy must

include stress management, treating underlying emotional issues, and self-care. You will acquire useful coping mechanisms through psychology and counseling-related approaches to handle any emotional obstacles that may come up along the way.

Self-Monitoring Techniques:

To avoid a relapse, self-monitoring measures are just as crucial to apply as a long-term maintenance strategy. With the help of these self-monitoring approaches, you will be able to keep tabs on your recovery and identify any little changes that might point to a recurrent infection. Among the self-monitoring strategies that work well are:

1. Maintaining a Symptom Diary: You can follow the patterns of your yeast infections and keep an eye on any changes in your body by keeping a thorough symptom journal. To help uncover patterns that may lead to recurrence, information regarding the degree of symptoms, the impact on daily activities, and any potential triggers should be recorded in this journal.

2. Regular pH Testing: Another good method to see any changes that can point to a yeast infection is to keep an eye on the pH of your vagina. With pre-made kits or pH test strips, performing a pH test at home is simple and convenient. You can see any deviations from the ideal range and take preventive steps to stop a full-blown infection by routinely checking your pH levels.

3. Regular Self-Examinations: An essential part of self-monitoring is being acquainted with your body and performing self-examinations on a regular basis. You can identify any yeast infections early on and treat them more effectively by keeping an eye out for any physical changes or subtle signs like itching, redness, or irregular discharge.

Regular Check-ups:

To maintain improvement and avoid recurrence, self-monitoring approaches must be used in conjunction with routine check-ups with your healthcare professional. Your entire health, including the health of your vagina, will be thoroughly assessed during these check-ups to make sure that any potential imbalances or risk factors are quickly found and taken care of. Your healthcare provider may do blood tests, perform a physical examination, and modify your treatment plan during these check-ups.

Research and Evidence-Based Practices:

I'm dedicated to giving you evidence-based, scientifically grounded techniques as a medical doctor and health and wellness coach. Studies have demonstrated that implementing these tactics into your self-monitoring routine and long-term maintenance strategy considerably lowers the chance of a recurrence of a yeast infection. You are controlling and avoiding future yeast infections in a proactive and thorough manner by following these procedures.

In summary, maintaining improvement and avoiding recurrence of yeast infections necessitates a team effort including lifestyle changes, self-monitoring methods, and routine examinations. By carefully putting these tactics into practise, you may give yourself the tools you need to effectively treat persistent yeast infections and take back authority over your health and wellbeing. Recall that you are not alone on this road, and you may become an expert in managing yeast infections with the help and advice of our team of professionals.

# Embracing Holistic Wellness

In the hectic and demanding world of today, we frequently neglect our health. We neglect to take a step back and evaluate our general well-being because we are too preoccupied with treating certain illnesses and problems, like yeast infections. I want to stress in this chapter the value of adopting a holistic perspective on wellness and the significant influence that taking care of our mental, emotional, and physical well-being can have on our general health.

First, let's clarify what holistic wellness entails. A holistic approach to wellbeing takes into account how our body, mind, and spirit are intertwined. It acknowledges that various facets of who we are are interconnected parts that impact one another rather than existing as distinct entities. Thus, we need to take care of every part of ourselves if we want to genuinely attain optimal health.

Many people make the mistake of treating their yeast infections only by treating their symptoms. To relieve the itching and discomfort, they take medication or apply topical lotions, but they neglect to treat the underlying reasons. This limited strategy frequently results in brief respite from the virus, but it eventually returns. By adopting a holistic approach to wellbeing, we can end this cycle and produce results that last.

Physical Well-being:
Treating the symptoms of a yeast infection is not the only aspect of taking care of our physical well-being. It entails being proactive in improving our general physical well-being. This entails taking up a nutritious diet, working out frequently, obtaining adequate rest, and maintaining proper hygiene.

A robust immune system is essential for preventing and combating yeast infections, and it can only be sustained by eating a balanced diet. We may encourage the growth of beneficial bacteria in our stomach, which helps to maintain a good balance of yeast and bacteria in our bodies, by include foods high in probiotics, such as yoghurt, sauerkraut, and kefir. Reducing the intake of processed carbs and sugar can also aid in starving the yeast and halting their expansion.

Engaging in regular exercise can strengthen our immune system and enhance blood circulation, which can facilitate the transportation of nutrients and oxygen to our cells. Additionally, it encourages the release of endorphins, which are organic mood enhancers that can lessen tension and anxiety.

Although it's sometimes forgotten, getting adequate sleep is crucial for maintaining our general health. Our bodies heal and regenerate as we sleep, which promotes the best possible performance of our immune system. Our immune systems can be weakened and we become more vulnerable to infections, including yeast infections, when we don't get enough sleep. As a result, making sleep a priority and creating a regular sleep routine are crucial.

Maintaining proper cleanliness is just another crucial part of taking care of our physical health. These behaviours serve to maintain a healthy balance of germs and prevent the overgrowth of yeast. They include keeping our genital area clean and dry, avoiding the use of strong soaps or douches, wearing breathable underwear and clothing, and changing out of damp or sweaty garments soon.

Mental Well-being:

Maintaining our general health also depends on our mental wellness. Our mentality, feelings, and thoughts have a big influence on our physical well-being. Weaknesses in our immune system, hormonal imbalance, and increased inflammation in our bodies can result from stress, anxiety, and negative thinking, which increases our vulnerability to yeast infections.

We must integrate stress management practises into our daily lives in order to support our mental health. This can involve routines like writing, yoga, deep breathing exercises, meditation, or just doing things that make us happy and calm. These techniques support inner serenity, lower stress levels, and mental calmness.

Stress management and the advancement of mental health might also benefit from counselling and psychology-related practises. Getting assistance from a holistically trained therapist or counsellor can teach us useful tools and techniques for stress management, emotion regulation, and developing an optimistic outlook.

Emotional Well-being:

The recognition, comprehension, and regulation of our emotions are all components of our emotional well-being. It entails creating constructive coping strategies and preserving wholesome interpersonal interactions. Our mental and physical health are intimately related to our emotional well-being, which is also essential for controlling yeast infections.

Taking care of ourselves emotionally is one thing we can do. This entails scheduling time for ourselves to engage in enjoyable and soothing activities. It might be as easy as reading a book, having a warm bath, engaging in a pastime, or spending time with close friends and family. By attending to our emotional needs, we can decompress and revitalise, which lowers stress and enhances general wellbeing.

Creating good coping mechanisms is also essential for handling the emotional difficulties that come with having a yeast infection. This can entail seeking out the assistance of friends, family, or support groups, practising self-compassion and forgiveness, creating boundaries, and learning how to communicate effectively.

In summary, adopting a holistic approach to wellbeing is critical to the thorough and long-term management of yeast infections. By taking care of our mental, emotional, and physical health, we may build an environment in our bodies that resists the expansion of yeast. It's critical to keep in mind that treating yeast infections involves more than just treating the symptoms; it also entails addressing the underlying causes and enhancing general health. We can improve our well-being and change our lives by taking a holistic approach.

# Self-Care Rituals for Ongoing Well-being

In the modern world, which is frequently hectic and stressful, it is more crucial than ever to look for ourselves. I have personal experience with the detrimental consequences of ignoring self-care as a physician and health coach. I hear concerns from a lot of individuals about feeling unbalanced, anxious, and overwhelmed. In an effort to care for others or fulfil the demands of their hectic lives, they frequently overlook their own needs. Numerous problems with physical, mental, and emotional health can result from this lack of self-care.

Self-care is vital to our general well-being and is not selfish. In order to be our best selves in every area of our lives, it is important that we take the time to nurture our bodies, brains, and spirits. It's about realising we are worthy of your time and effort. Making self-care a priority helps us manage stress, avoid burnout, and live more satisfying lives.

What then does self-care actually include in daily life? Since everyone of us has distinct wants and preferences, it might imply different things to different individuals. The secret is to engage in pursuits and routines that make you happy, content, and feel refreshed. Here are some doable suggestions for self-care routines you can do on a regular basis:

1. Mindful Breathing: Our wellbeing can be greatly enhanced by setting aside a little period of time each day to concentrate on our breathing. We can feel more at peace and present when we practise mindful breathing, which also helps to clear our minds and lower stress. Locate a peaceful area, settle into a comfortable position, and inhale and exhale slowly while paying attention to the sensation of the breath entering and exiting your body.

2. Daily Movement: Frequent physical activity is beneficial for our mental and emotional health in addition to its benefits for our physical health. Choose hobbies or pastimes you love to engage in, such as

walking, yoga, dancing, or sports. The secret is to move in a way that makes you happy and content.

3. Nourishing Nutrition: Providing our bodies with wholesome nourishment is a type of self-care. Consider the nutritional value of the food you eat and select nutrient-dense selections that promote your general health. Consume a diet rich in whole grains, fruits, vegetables, lean meats, and healthy fats. Drink lots of water throughout the day to stay hydrated as well.

4. Quality Sleep: Sleeping well and getting enough of it is essential for maintaining our general health and wellbeing. Create a calming evening ritual that enables you to unwind and get your body and mind ready for slumber. Keep your bedroom cold, dark, and quiet to create a conducive sleeping environment. To encourage better sleep, put away electronic gadgets an hour before bed and engage in relaxing exercises like deep breathing or meditation.

5. Creative Expression: Taking up artistic endeavours can be a potent self-care strategy. Choose hobbies that let you express yourself and release your creative energy, whether it's writing, painting, playing an instrument, or cooking. Engaging in these activities can lower stress, improve mood, and give one a sense of contentment and success.

6. Time in Nature: It has been demonstrated that time spent in nature enhances mood, lowers stress levels, and enhances general wellbeing. Whether it's strolling through a park, hiking through the woods, or just relaxing in a garden, make it a point to spend time outside. Enjoy the sights, sounds, and scents of the natural world and let yourself feel rooted and connected.

7. Self-Reflection and Journaling: One crucial aspect of self-care is reflecting on our feelings, ideas, and experiences. Schedule frequent times to reflect on yourself, either by writing in a journal or by just being still. Take advantage of this time to reflect on your actions and routines, as well as to check in with yourself and explore your feelings.

8. Social Connection: Since we are social creatures, taking care of our relationships is an essential component of self-care. Spend quality time with your loved ones by engaging in activities together, having frequent phone conversations, or going on coffee dates. Those who cheer you on, support you, and infuse your life with happiness and enthusiasm are the individuals you should be around.

These are but a few suggestions to get you going on your path of self-care. Recall that there is no one-size-fits-all strategy for self-care. Finding what works for you and giving it attention in your life are the key points. Be kind to yourself, be consistent, and start small. Self-care is a continuous process that calls for self-compassion, dedication, and intention.

Including self-care practises in your daily routine will improve not only your personal health but also the health of people around you. Taking care of ourselves makes it easier for us to be there for others, carry out our obligations, and lead purposeful, fulfilling lives.

Make self-care a top priority and an indisputable aspect of your everyday routine. Your spirit, mind, and body will all appreciate it. Never forget that you are worth the expenditure.

# Celebrating Personal Growth and Resilience

Taking care of yeast infections can be difficult and irritating at times. To enhance your health, you must be committed, patient, and willing to make the required adjustments. The fact that you have progressed this far already shows how resilient and determined you are. The first step toward living a better life has been made, and this is something to be proud of and acknowledged.

Honoring personal development and resiliency is crucial because it recognises the effort and diligence you have dedicated to looking after yourself. It serves as a reminder that you are able to overcome obstacles and accomplish your objectives. By acknowledging your accomplishments, you are validating your path and rewarding yourself.

Honoring resilience and personal development is also a source of inspiration and drive. Recognizing our accomplishments gives us more self-assurance and motivates us to keep going. It enables us to meet upcoming problems with resiliency and resolve by serving as a reminder of our skills and talents.

Studies have indicated that acknowledging and appreciating our individual development and adaptability enhances our general state of wellbeing. According to a study by psychologist Dr. Barbara Fredrickson, feeling happy, proud, and grateful can broaden our perspectives and strengthen our inner resources. We are fostering happy feelings that can strengthen our ability to handle stress, strengthen our bonds with others, and generally improve our quality of life when we celebrate our accomplishments.

So how can we honour our individual development and fortitude while we navigate the management of yeast infections? Here are some recommendations:

1. Reflect on your progress: Think back on how much progress you have made since beginning to treat your yeast infection. Consider the adjustments you have made, the difficulties you have surmounted, and the knowledge you have gained. Share your thoughts with a friend or family member who can offer support, or write them down in a journal. This will remind you of your tenacity and resolve while also assisting you in celebrating your accomplishments.

2. Reward yourself: Reward yourself with something special to acknowledge your efforts and advancements. It could be as easy as taking a soothing bath, eating your favourite food, or taking the day off to do something you enjoy. Seek opportunities to practise self-love and self-care; these are crucial for preserving your wellbeing.

3. Share your success: Telling others about your storey will help you celebrate your resilience and personal development. By sharing your experience, you boost your own self-confidence and serve as an inspiration to others who might be going through something similar. To meet people and share your experiences, consider creating a blog or joining online forums or support groups.

4. Practice gratitude: Develop an attitude of thankfulness for the advancements you have achieved. Spend a few minutes every day remembering the good things that have happened in your life and feeling thankful for the possibilities for development, the lessons discovered, and the support you have had. Your perspective can change from one of dissatisfaction and negativity to one of appreciation and optimism with the aid of gratitude.

5. Set new goals: Honoring personal development and resiliency requires not only reflecting on the past but also looking to the future. Establish new objectives for yourself and use your accomplishments as motivation to keep going. You can continue your journey of growth and resilience by setting objectives to incorporate healthy behaviours into your lifestyle, enhance your self-care routine, or research new treatment choices.

Recall that treating yeast infections requires adopting a complete approach to wellbeing in addition to looking for a fast cure. In addition to recognising your accomplishments, you are also promoting your general wellbeing when you celebrate your perseverance and personal growth. Honor your strength, enjoy your path, and keep developing and prospering. You possess the ability to overcome obstacles and design a healthier life for yourself.

Milton Keynes UK
Ingram Content Group UK Ltd.
UKHW020644201123
432908UK00019B/2554